Maximize Your Workouts

Achieve the Body You Have Always Wanted by Implementing the Fitness and Diet Secrets That All Top Trainers Live by

D & R Health and Fitness Group

TABLE OF CONTENTS

INTRODUCTION

One of my closest friends, Amy, has always struggled with her fitness. She was the kind of person who always hopped on the latest trend, either for her diet or how she exercised. If she heard some new shortcut or health tip, she would immediately adopt it. It didn't matter whether she was given this information by a friend, if she found it in a magazine, or if she heard it from a so-called 'fitness expert' who she met at the gym. If there was a new fad diet, she would follow it for a few weeks before giving up. She had tried CrossFit, Zumba classes, and just about every other new training fad. She read through magazines and bought every protein powder, slimming tea, and fat-burning pills that were recommended to her.

Despite her efforts, Amy never saw lasting results. Her goals were always to lose weight and build her strength and fitness. She would occasionally lose weight before immediately putting it back on again the moment she stopped whatever diet or fitness fad she was following. Amy also never seemed to feel any fitter; she moved so quickly from one fitness program to the next that she never felt progress because she either didn't have a reference for comparison or because she had not kept with the diet or program long enough for any notable changes to have been made.

Many of you might have been through something similar to Amy's story. Whether you have been through a million training fads, or are just overwhelmed about which one to pick, it is something a lot of people struggle with.

It can be hard to know where to start when it comes to getting fit. There are so many different "truths" about fitness that have floated around throughout the years. The number of fitness fads that come and go, as well as all the fallacies they contain, may seem like one of life's constants. It seems that there is always some new and true way to exercise that will help you reach your goals. Because we are so engaged with all different kinds of media every day, we are constantly attacked with new diets that will magically lead you to weight loss or better results in the gym. We are told we need every supplement and protein powder possible, that we won't see results unless we are overloaded with them, following a very specific diet and training schedule.

However, none of this is true. There is no quick fix diet or highly specific workout that you need to follow in order to gain muscle, lose fat, and develop your strength. Furthermore, no protein powder or health bar is going to make you stronger and healthier unless incorporated into a balanced lifestyle. The key to reaching your full fitness potential is through balancing your diet and maximizing your workouts. Your workouts do not need to

be complex and constantly changing for you to see results (although, changing it up sometimes can be helpful). You will see the best results and continual progress by being consistent with what you are doing and by being more mindful and deliberate with how you work out. This book will guide you through the best ways to do that.

It doesn't matter what stage of your fitness journey you find yourself in, this book will be beneficial for you. If you are just starting out, this book will give you a comprehensive guide of where to start and how to get results immediately. You will not have to spend months trying all the different workouts and eating guides to find out what works for you. By following the tips and tricks provided in this book, you are sidestepping all that white noise and you will be able to see progress in a matter of weeks instead of months or possibly years.

If you are a few years into your fitness journey, this book will be just as helpful for you. It is natural to start to stagnate after a few years of any type of training. Maybe you have never seen the results you wanted, even after years of consistent training. Or maybe you feel that your training has started to feel stale, that you no longer feel challenged, or that you are not progressing. We will provide you with new ways to work out, as well as ways to get the most out of your current workouts.

Sometimes it is more important to train smarter than it is to train harder. Through these tips, you will find yourself enjoying your workouts again, and more importantly, thriving as your level of fitness and strength steadily increase. Maximizing your workouts is an invaluable skill to learn at any part of your fitness journey because you should always be pushing yourself beyond your limits and what you think you are capable of.

You may be wondering what makes me qualified to guide you through this process - what expertise do I have that is a cut above the rest? The simple answer is experience and passion. I have been involved in the health and fitness industry for over a decade. I have a Bachelors in Science for Health and Physical Education; so I have 5 years of studying to back up my understanding of fitness. I have also competed in bodybuilding shows and have been a personal trainer for both male and female clients. Through their nutrition and workouts, we reached their fitness goals. I have also been on both sides—both being trained and helping others train. This makes me uniquely qualified not only to guide you, but also to understand what you are going through as you work towards your goals.

I have also been in the exact same position as you before. Even the fittest people have started at the beginning or found themselves in slumps where they are not at the level of fitness and strength they want to be. Having gone through that frustration myself, I am passionate about helping people past that point and helping them to get to the level they have always dreamt of. I used the techniques from this book to get to the physique I currently have, which is

the one I have always dreamed of. I am stronger than I have ever been, and more importantly, I feel completely confident and capable with my body and what it is able to do. I have tried almost every route to fitness, and I have found this to be the most efficient—and sustainable—way to find your ideal fitness lifestyle. Lastly, and perhaps most importantly, I am passionate about fitness and about helping people to reach their peak. I have dedicated years to nutrition and fitness, to find the best routes to it, and to helping people be their best selves.

This book will provide the ultimate guide for getting the most out of your workouts. First and foremost, it will outline the ideal diet to follow to maximize your fitness potential. Food is how we fuel our body, and it is the part of our fitness that we have to work at throughout the entire day. We will then dive into the benefits of focusing on the mind-to-muscle connection, what it is and why it is so important to your progress. This involves focusing on being fully controlled with your reps and focusing on how each exercise works the specific muscle or body part that it is targeting. You will also be introduced to all the different kinds of training, ranging from strength to endurance training, the benefits of each, and how to implement them. You will also be taught how to build your own workouts, as well as how to continually spice up and change your workouts to see the best results. We will also look at the importance of cardio and the different ways that you can introduce it into your weekly workout schedule. And we can't forget the importance of rest days for muscle recovery and the role of supplements in your fitness regime.

You will finish this book feeling fully informed and more than capable of tackling every aspect of your fitness journey, armed with all the knowledge and guidance you could need. Your days of struggling with different workouts and diets have come to an end. This will become your definitive guide for fitness, for developing and maintaining your ideal physique, and for finding the true limits of your strength.

CHAPTER 1: THE IMPORTANCE OF GOOD NUTRITION

You may be asking yourself why a book focused on workouts would start out with a chapter on nutrition. Well, it's because one of the biggest mistakes people make when they are trying to get fit is ignoring what they are eating. People might feel that because they have had an intense and sweaty two-hour session at the gym in the morning, they are able to eat anything they want for the rest of the day. They might feel that it is justified because they have 'burnt it off.' This is a common misconception and is one of the main reasons people struggle to lose weight and reach their peak level of fitness.

In some ways, your diet plays a far bigger role in your physical health and physique than lifting or other forms of exercise do. You may work out a few times a week, but your diet is something you have to pay attention to 24/7. From the moment you wake up to the moment you go to sleep, you are making decisions about what you are going to eat and drink. Several times a day you have to decide between healthy or unhealthy choices.

Furthermore, if you are aiming to lose weight, it is nearly impossible to do that entirely through exercise. To lose weight, you need to be in a calorie deficit, which means that you have to take in fewer calories than you burn. While working out certainly does burn calories, it takes a ton more effort to burn 500–700 calories in a day through exercise rather than simply cutting it out from your diet. This also means that you can unintentionally be taking in more calories than you are burning if you are not watching what you eat (Gomez, 2016). So, you might be working out hard and consistently, but not seeing changes to your body, or maybe even gaining weight. This is because you are eating more than you are burning.

You've probably heard the old adage that 'abs are made in the kitchen.' In other words, your muscle definition is dependent more on what you eat than what you lift. But how true is this? Let's look into it. The appearance of your abdominal muscles is determined by three factors: genetics, muscularity, and body fat percentage. Your genetics determine the shape of your abs; your muscularity determines how big they are and your body fat percentage determines whether they are visible (Lecompte, 2016). Everyone has these muscles, and they can be incredibly muscular and strong but still hidden. It does not matter how muscular your abdominal muscles are if they are hidden beneath a layer of fat because you are not watching your diet. Therefore, the key to getting your ideal physique, whether it is muscular or toned, is through your diet, as well as how you exercise. You are not going to achieve your goals by doing 100 crunches every day, you are going to achieve them through following a balanced and nutrient-dense diet.

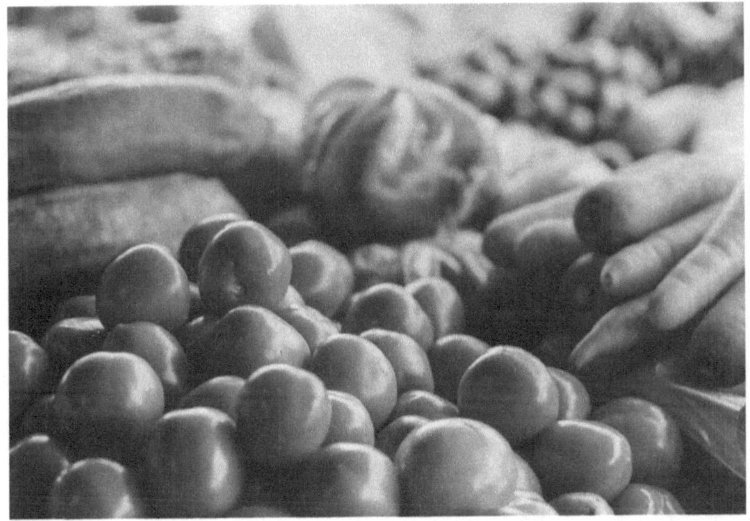

Nutrition is also important because of the energy and stamina it can give us for our physical fitness. The different nutrients and macros we gain from our food aid us in different ways and give us different amounts of energy. For example, think about how you feel after you have a bowl of oats versus how you feel after a bowl of sugary cereal. You are far more likely to feel full and energized after eating oats, and sluggish and unsatisfied after eating the sugary cereal. Oats are complex carbohydrates which means they break down slowly and keep you full for hours. They are also full of antioxidants and nutrients. On the other hand, sugary cereals are simple and high-sugar carbohydrates.

They break down quickly, giving you a burst of energy but then causing you to dip and feel lethargic. Therefore, if you were going to work out, you should opt for the oats, not only because they are healthier, but also because they are more nutrient-dense and will enable you to have the best workout possible.

If you are aiming for fat loss, there are a few ways you should structure your diet. As previously mentioned, staying in a calorie deficit is the only way to lose weight. However, counting calories can be tiresome and hard to maintain every day. Fortunately, there are ways to eat that allow you to stay in a calorie deficit without having to specifically count calories.

One of the first ways is to cut out all processed sugar. We have access to so much more sugary foods and snacks than we ever have before. Think back to the last time you went to the supermarket, and maybe found your way down the cereal aisle. While there may have been a few healthier options, you might have noticed that 90% of the selection was filled with cookie cereal, or chocolate and peanut butter-flavored puffs. If you went down the candy and chocolate aisle, you might have noticed the same. There are so many sugar-filled treats available in our modern society, and these endless options are why over 70% of adults in the United States of America are overweight or obese (Chen, 2018). Sugar is added to so many of the foods we buy every day and many people do not tend to realize it. It is also often added to foods that we don't expect because they aren't sweet, such as savory crackers or even premade pasta sauces. Foods filled with sugar, such as sweets, chips, chocolates, pastries, or anything highly processed, are very high in calories. They are also low in nutrients, vitamins, and minerals, or anything else that is actually useful to your body. All this sugar becomes stored as fat and causes you to gain weight. Also, despite these foods being high in calories, they are often not satisfying and do not keep you full. Therefore, you are going to end up eating an excessive amount to feel satisfied or resort to eating more of other foods. Either will cause your body to store fat and gain weight (Medicine Plus, 2021). Cutting out sugar and processed foods is essential for fat loss.

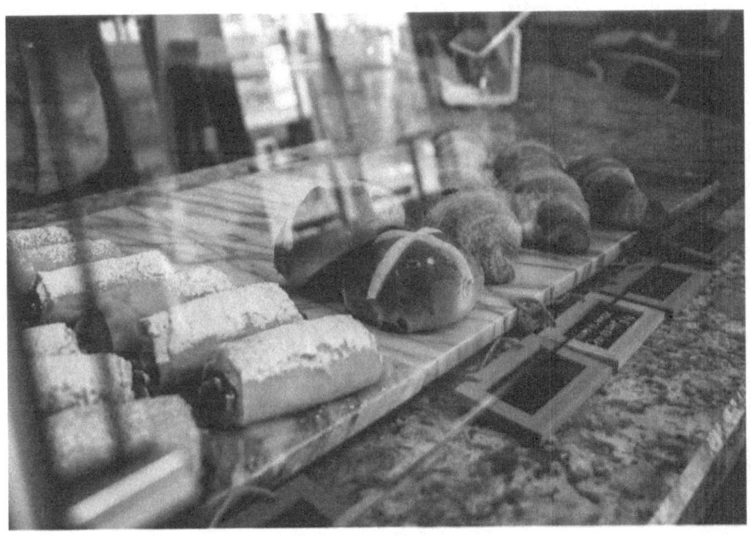

While it is essential to cut down on sweets, chips, and baked goods, another way to avoid added sugar in your diet is to cook more at home. This allows you to know exactly what is going into your food. Make your own pasta sauce instead of buying it in jars. Make oats from scratch instead of buying flavored instant oats to which you just add water. All of these will make a significant dent in your sugar intake, and therefore help you to lose weight.

Another tip for losing fat is to cut out eating carbohydrates late at night. Not only does this cause fat gain, but it also stifles muscle growth. Carbohydrates, especially simple ones, such as sugary snacks and chocolate, break down into sugar in your body and therefore cause your blood sugar levels to spike. This produces high levels of insulin in your blood, which can disrupt the muscle-repair process that your body undergoes overnight. Sleep is an essential time for your body to perform self-restoration (Comite, 2013). Furthermore, if you eat carbohydrates late at night, you are not burning them off. If you eat carbs earlier in the day, you are active enough to use them and the energy they provide. However, if you are going straight to sleep, those carbohydrates are not being used up and are converted to fat and stored in your body. In order to stimulate fat loss, aim to stop eating any form of carbohydrates after your dinner. One of the worst culprits is alcohol, as beverages like beer and wine are very high in carbohydrates. Beer has one of the highest glycemic values of any beverage (Comite, 2013). It also helps to avoid snacks such as chips and popcorn, and desserts like ice creams or cake.

Another important—and often overlooked—factor in weight loss is how hydrated you are. Drinking enough water is essential for your health in general. Water benefits your workouts, your sleep, and your general energy levels. There are several reasons why water is beneficial for weight loss. Firstly, if you are currently drinking juice, sodas, and alcohol, replacing those with water will greatly reduce your daily calorie intake, which will help you to lose weight. Most fruit juices and sodas are filled with sugar and are high in calories, however, they do not fill you up or provide much—if any—nutritional value. These are known as 'empty calories' and could be better spent on foods that fill you up and provide you with vitamins and minerals. Water has zero calories and is a far better choice that will help you to lose weight.

It is also pretty common to mistake thirst for hunger, and so people tend to reach for more food instead of a glass of water. By drinking water consistently, you are less likely to do that. Drinking water has been shown to be a natural appetite suppressant. When the stomach is full, the brain is signaled to stop eating. By drinking water, you are able to fill up your stomach, which leads to you feeling full and satisfies your hunger signals. Drinking water has even been shown to burn calories. Studies have shown that drinking cold water increases your energy expenditure and you are more likely to burn 2–3% more calories than usual in the hour and a half after you drink cold water (Huizen, 2018). Water is also a necessary component for burning fat; without it, the body cannot properly metabolize carbs and your stored fat. Therefore, drinking water allows your body to burn off fat.

Water is also key for successful workouts. Drinking sufficient water is essential for the healthy functioning of our organs and allows your muscles, joints, and connective tissues to move correctly. It also prevents dehydration, which becomes a risk when doing intense workouts (Bjarnadottir, 2017). The benefits of drinking water are endless, both for fat loss, as well as your general health. The recommended amount is between 1.5 to 2 liters a day. To achieve that, you should constantly have a water bottle on hand so that you can sip on it throughout the day.

One of the last actions necessary for fat loss is getting enough sleep—and being consistent with the time in which you sleep! Many people underestimate the importance of sleep and how much your body does while you are out cold. Studies suggest that insufficient sleep is one of the common causes of weight gain and is also linked to a higher body mass index. A lack of sleep can lead to increased secretion of the stress hormone, cortisol, which is linked to weight gain because of the stress it puts your body under (Pullen, 2017). People who suffer from poor sleep also tend to consume more calories. This can be due to the increased stress caused by sleep deprivation, or even being awake later, and therefore more prone to snack later and more frequently. A lack of sleep also affects your ability to make good food choices and fight cravings. Sleep deprivation dulls the frontal lobe of the brain, which is where decisions are made. Therefore, you will struggle to make good ones if you are not getting enough sleep. It has also been found that food as a reward stimulates the brain more when you haven't slept well. This will affect your ability to practice self-control. Lastly, sleep affects your resting metabolic rate, which is essentially how many calories you burn when you are at rest. Sleep deprivation can lower your metabolic rate, meaning you burn fewer calories, and are therefore more likely to gain weight. Your workouts will also be negatively affected by lack of sleep, as you won't have the energy to give it your all.

So, sleep is vital to fat loss and your overall health. Your ideal amount of sleep depends on your age, level of activity, as well as simply the number of hours you feel you need to function at your best. The recommended amount of sleep for adults is between 7 and 10 hours every night. Some people are sluggish if they sleep any longer than 7 hours, while others will need the full 10 hours of sleep. This is especially true if you are very active, as your body needs time to rest and recover. It is also essential that you sleep at roughly the same time every night. This allows you to fall asleep and wake up more easily, maximizing your sleeping hours and allowing your body as much time as possible to rest. For example, perhaps you can aim to go to sleep at 10 p.m. every night and wake up at 6 a.m. every morning. For the best results, you should do this every night—even on the weekends when it is a lot harder to stick to.

If the words 'Banting' or 'Atkins' mean anything to you, you are probably aware of the early 2000s dieting craze that vilified carbs for the general public. Suddenly, bread and potatoes went from being the staple of many diets to being the enemy that was creating your belly. You might have fallen into the trap yourself, or knew friends or family members that were suddenly making cauliflower into pizza bases. There have been a number of diets over the years that shun the consumption of carbohydrates as something that causes you to gain fat. After Banting, people went for the keto diet, which encouraged consumption of high fat and protein with zero carbohydrates. However, while there are some simple and sugary carbohydrates that might be wise to avoid in the name of health, without any carbohydrates, your diet is unbalanced, and you would be missing out on many benefits by avoiding them.

While you should avoid eating simple carbs and avoid eating all carbs late at night, carbohydrates are our greatest source of energy, and we would be unable to maximize the way we workout without them. Our body breaks down the carbs we eat into glucose, which is used for energy for our cells. If you are doing an hour of exercise, for example, you will need carbohydrates to fuel it, such as white rice or my personal favorite, a sweet potato pre-workout. If you are doing more than an hour of aerobic exercise, you may need carbs during your workout to keep you going. This can be in the form of a carb supplement powder or an apple intra-workout. You also need to eat carbohydrates after your workout in order to replenish the energy lost in your muscles during the workout (Medicine Plus, 2021). Without carbohydrates, you will feel lethargic during your workouts and it will take longer for your muscles to recover and develop afterward. Your overall performance will suffer, and you will not see the progress that you want.

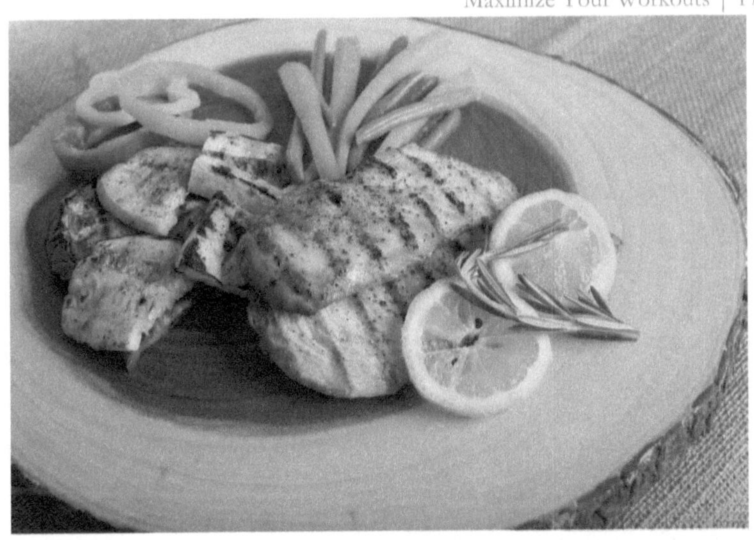

Carbohydrates are important for the inner workings of your body too—the stuff that you won't be concerned with until it stops working. You need carbohydrates in your diet to fuel your major organs, regulate your digestive system, and keep your cholesterol levels in check. Carbohydrates help to fuel all of your organs, such as your brain, your kidneys, your heart, and your central nervous system. You will also get the necessary fiber for your body from eating carbs, as fiber is a complex healthy carbohydrate. Your body cannot digest fiber, it simply continues through the intestines and stimulates digestion (Cleveland Clinic, 2014). It is important for your digestive system to function optimally because it is how your body takes in all the nutrients from the foods you are eating. It doesn't matter what you're eating if your gut isn't working well enough to absorb it. Carbs are therefore essential for maintaining the balance and function of your gut. Fiber is also responsible for keeping your cholesterol levels low.

So, what kinds of carbs should you be eating? It is important to go for complex carbs over simple carbs, so opt for sweet potato, brown rice, and bulgur wheat over normal potatoes, white rice, and regular pasta. Complex carbs contain more fiber, as well as nutrients, and take longer to break down and release energy into your body. This means you will be fuller and more energized for longer. Other versions of healthy carbohydrate-rich foods include fruits, such as berries, apples, pears, and bananas. Legumes are also a good source of carbs, particularly lentils, chickpeas, and black beans. It is important that you include carbs in your diet every day to fuel yourself and feel your best.

While carbohydrates are key for your best diet, protein is just as important. Protein is an essential component for our cells to replicate themselves, and therefore helps in creating the building blocks that make up our body. Protein is a macronutrient, meaning our body needs a lot of it. Our bodies also do not store protein; therefore, you need to eat protein daily; in appropriate amounts and in correctly spaced apart meals in order for it to fully benefit your body.

The primary function of protein is building. Protein is made up of long chains called amino acids. The cells in your body use amino acids to repair themselves and to replicate. Therefore, protein is essential for muscle recovery, as well as muscle development. It is also important in building your bones, cartilage, and skin. Your hair and nails are mostly made up of protein. Protein is also necessary for distributing oxygen throughout your body, as your red blood cells create a protein compound responsible for this. It is an essential component for your body to regulate hormones and digestion. Also, approximately half of the protein that you consume goes into making digestive enzymes (Piedmont Healthcare, 2019).

Eating a high-protein diet is particularly important in terms of working out. It speeds up your recovery time for your muscles in between training and does the same if you happen to injure yourself. It is also essential for building muscle—if you do not eat protein, what is your body meant to build muscle out of? It helps to reduce the risk of losing muscle and helps to build lean muscle. Eating a significant amount of protein also helps to maintain your weight and lose fat—it keeps you full and therefore stops you from reaching for unhealthy, high-calorie foods. It curbs hunger but also gives us all the nutrients we need.

There are a ton of whole foods that provide a significant amount of protein for your daily diet. You can get it from lean meats such as chicken, turkey, and lamb. Fish is also an excellent source of protein, especially lean fish, such as cod and halibut, and fatty fish, such as salmon and herring. Other good sources of protein are eggs and dairy products, particularly greek yogurt. There are also plant-based options to give your diet some variation—most notably, nuts, seeds, and legumes. You can eat the nuts whole, such as walnuts, almonds, and pine nuts, or eat nut butters, such as peanut butter or almond butter. You can try sunflower, sesame, and pumpkin seeds, perhaps topping your morning oatmeal with them. High-protein legumes include chickpeas, lentils, and tofu. You can also opt to add protein powders and protein bars to your diet for an extra kick of protein. This can be especially helpful on days when you're working out. It is highly beneficial to consume protein within thirty minutes of a workout, and a good way to do this is with a protein shake or a protein smoothie. This kickstarts muscle recovery. There are a number of options for adding a variety of protein-rich foods into your diet every day, and it is imperative that you do!

One of the last things we will look at in regards to nutrition is the essential vitamins that your body needs to function optimally. Our body requires vitamins and minerals to function every day, as they perform vital roles in the maintenance of our body. Vitamins and minerals help the body repair and reproduce cells. They help the blood cells to carry oxygen and nutrients around the body, and they create the chemical messengers that travel around your body controlling your hormones and your organs. They are invaluable to the healthy functioning of your body. There are around 30 vitamins and minerals that your body requires to function but that it does not make enough of on its own (Harvard Health, 2018). Vitamins are micronutrients, meaning we only need small amounts of them.

There are several vitamins you need for everyday living, but as you get more active, there are specific vitamins that will benefit your fitness journey. Some of these include calcium, magnesium, iron, zinc, and vitamins B, C, and D (Culp, 2015).

Calcium is important for your bones; it helps to repair, maintain, and grow them. Calcium also helps with the regulation of muscle contraction, nerve conduction, and blood clotting. Magnesium is important for energy, as it is essential in metabolizing macronutrients in your body, such as protein, fats, and carbohydrates. Magnesium deficiency is usually characterized by low energy and fatigue and can severely impact your endurance training if not corrected. Iron is an essential supplement for any active person, and it has been found that endurance athletes require approximately 70% more iron in their diet than the average person. Iron deficiency can impair muscle function and is linked to fatigue and severe lack of energy. Zinc regulates our metabolic function, and if we are deficient it could lead to easy weight gain. It also aids in the growth and repair of muscle tissue, regulation of the immune system, and energy production. Vitamins such as B, C, and D are essential for maintaining optimal cell health.

As you can see, vitamins and minerals are invaluable for developing and maintaining fitness. While these vitamins are available in your foods, you can also take supplements to ensure that you are getting the optimal level of each in your diet.

The best way to eat is to find a balanced and sustainable diet, full of macros, nutrients, and vitamins that nourish your body and aid in building your muscles. Balance is important because everything has a purpose; everything you eat provides something your body needs that it cannot get anywhere else. If you do not focus on your nutrition, you will never be able to reach the peak of your fitness potential. Everything you do in the gym is based on the foundation of what you put into your body in the kitchen. It is therefore essential that you are eating a balanced diet, getting enough carbs and proteins, and cutting down on sugar-filled processed foods. This is the only way to lose fat, gain and maintain muscle, and develop your ideal physique.

CHAPTER 2: HOW TO FIND YOUR MIND-TO-MUSCLE CONNECTION

Think back to the last time you worked out and the last time you were lifting weights. I want you to try to remember what you were thinking about throughout your workout. Were you focusing on each rep, slowly and deliberating feeling the strain on your body? Or was your mind wandering as you absent-mindedly went through the motions? Maybe you were looking at someone else at the gym? Maybe you were thinking about what you were going to eat after your workout? Maybe your mind was just not there at all. This is natural but it is also one of the most significant reasons why you are not seeing the results that you want.

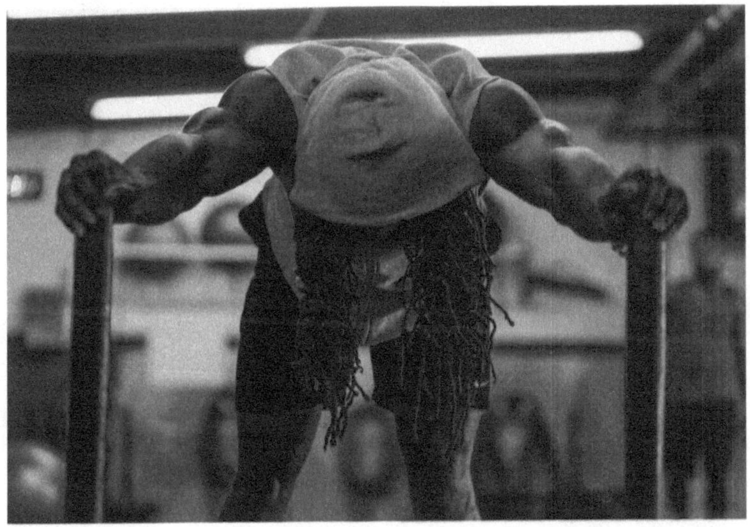

One of the biggest mistakes we make when working out is not connecting our minds to what we are doing. If we are mindless and simply trying to get through the exercise rather than focusing on how it is working us, we are often not training to the best of our ability.

This is where the mind-to-muscle connection comes in. It is about establishing a connection with your muscles when you work out instead of just going through the motions. It is also about blocking out any external factors that may distract you—maybe that's the noise of the gym around you or the other people near you. By filtering these out, you work out better. Studies have shown that this mindful engagement results in a far more effective workout and that thinking deliberately about working a targeted muscle can exercise it without you even moving it (Opler, 2019). While this sounds crazy, trials have shown that it can be true.

The Ohio University Heritage College of Osteopathic Medicine conducted an experiment whereby they wrapped the wrists of 29 participants in a cast for 4 weeks. Half of the participants were instructed to sit quietly for 11 minutes a day, five times a week, and visualize flexing their immobile wrist. The other half were told to do nothing. When the cast was taken off 4 weeks later, it was found that the visualization group's wrists were twice as strong as the other group who had done nothing (Clark et al., 2014). This demonstrates the power our mind has in developing the strength of our body. The greatest mistake you can make is underestimating that power and not utilizing it when trying to reach your peak physical form.

The mind-to-muscle connection is also essential because it helps you to isolate the muscles you are working on and ensures that your form is correct. You want to put yourself in a position where you are able to achieve perfect form. You should be feeling it mostly in the muscle you are targeting. For example, if you are exercising your back, your arms should not be getting fatigued before your back. This is a sure sign that your form is incorrect, and you are not focusing on targeting the right muscles.

So how does one develop the mind-to-muscle connection? This is not something that you achieve in one workout or in one day. Fostering this connection is a process. It is something that you have to focus on doing over weeks and months. In time, it will become habitual, something that you don't even realize you are doing. It will become second nature. But until that time, it needs to be something you are constantly working at improving. You will want to start with lighter weights than you usually would. They should still be heavy enough that your muscles feel fatigued at the end of 12 reps. However, by using slightly lighter weights, you can focus more on your muscles rather than just getting through the reps and being forced to cheat by assisting with secondary muscles. It also allows you to have more control with each rep, which helps you to feel the muscles as they are working.

Another trick is to lift with your eyes closed as you begin to form this connection. By shutting your eyes, you can try to visualize the muscles you are targeting and block out the distractions around you. You should be cautious lifting with your eyes closed if you have balance problems or are doing an exercise that requires you to see what you are doing. You should also make sure that you are not lifting too heavily—although, you shouldn't be lifting heavy, anyway, if you are trying to develop your mind-to-muscle connection. Another trick that may help you to develop the connection is to have your workout partner touch the area that you are trying to hit. Feeling that physical touch on the muscle you are trying to work out naturally links the brain to that muscle.

These are two sure-fire ways to get your mind into the right headspace, but you may experiment and find others that work for you.

It is also important to start with isolation exercises first and master those before moving on to compound movements. It will be far easier to master if you only have one muscle to focus on instead of several. As you find this technique coming more naturally to you, you can then move on to compound movements and test your limits by seeing if you can work on multiple muscles at once.

It is also essential that you warm up before you begin lifting. While this is always true, it is especially helpful when trying to build a mind-to-muscle connection. Warming up increases blood flow to the muscles and increases flexibility. It gives your body a chance to get ready for workouts and decreases the risk of injuries. The increased blood flow to your muscles will often help you to build a mind-to-muscle connection (Saini, 2020). To warm up for resistance training, you should stretch out, focusing on the muscle groups and joints you are going to target. It might also be helpful to do 10–15 minutes of light cardio to warm up. It is a way of priming your body for the workout and helping you to connect.

It is also important to focus on the eccentric portion of each rep just as much as the concentric portion. The eccentric part of a rep is also known as the negative work of a lift. It is the part where you are lowering the weight after having lifted it. In these movements, your muscles are being lengthened as well as stretched. Most people make the mistake of focusing on the lift part of the rep and not the lowering. They will expend all their energy pulling the weight up, and then relax their muscles and just let it drop. This is a huge mistake I see many people make all the time at the gym. Studies have shown that the eccentric portion of a rep causes more muscle growth than concentric-only training. In fact, eccentric moves can actually create significantly more growth, as the muscle is producing 25–50% more force during the eccentric part of a lift than during the concentric (Ottinger, 2019). When you get to the top of your lift, hold it there for a few seconds and focus on squeezing your muscles as hard as physically possible. This contraction will help stimulate muscle growth. Furthermore, it will help you to feel and pinpoint the muscle you are working on. Then, instead of dropping the weight, lower it slowly. You can even count this movement out, making sure that you take at least 2 - 5 seconds to get back to your starting point. By doing this, you never allow the muscle to relax during your reps. It will help you to foster your mind-to-muscle connection because you will constantly be paying attention to the muscle you are working. By doing this, you will see the most improvement in your muscles and your strength.

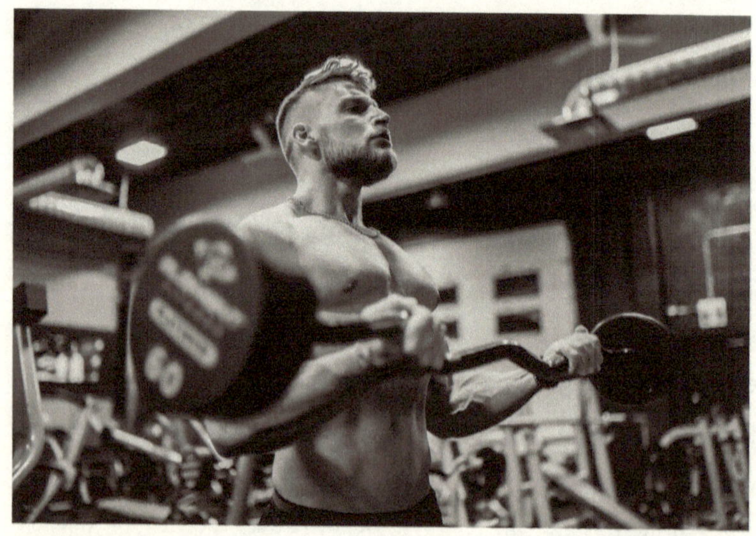

Now, let's dive into how to achieve this connection with the different muscle groups. For each group, there are different ways to connect your mind to the muscle, and different tricks that might make the development of this connection easier.

First, let us start with the back. The muscles of the back are extremely important and often ignored. Often people focus on their abs but don't develop their backs, which causes an imbalance and can lead to injury. Plus, a strong back is so important for all areas of fitness and everyday life.

Some people find it difficult to focus on this large area, but there are a few tips that can help you to truly hone in on working your back muscles. One of the best pieces of advice you will ever get is to picture your hands as hooks that are just holding the weight, as if your arm was cut off at the elbow. Therefore, when you move, you should be pulling your arms back with your back, and not bending the hooks. Your forearms, hands, and wrists should be in a fixed position. Perfecting this form is the key to maximizing your back workouts.

Another tip is to focus on how you are controlling your shoulder blades, or scapula, when you are lifting. Many of the muscles you move in your back assist in moving your shoulder blades too. Therefore, they serve as a good focus point to guide your mind to the muscle that you are actually working. If you are unable to control your shoulder blades when lifting, your back muscles will be unable to function at their peak and thus will not develop at the rate that you expect (Schepis, 2019).

When exercising your back, it is important to focus on both your scapula retraction and elevation. Retraction is being able to move your shoulder blades forward and back, while elevation is moving them up and down, almost in a shrugging motion. Mastering both is key to truly engaging your back and building strength in these important muscles. An easy way to achieve this with out overthinking it is to puff your chest up and pinch your shoulder blades together.

Next, let us look at the chest. The chest is arguably one of the hardest muscle groups to achieve the mind-to-muscle connection with, and many people struggle with this part of the body, especially when they're beginners to lifting. If you are having trouble developing this connection, sometimes it helps to start off with your chest first thing before jumping into anything else. It may also be beneficial to get a small pump on your pecs before you start. You can do this by doing any of your usual chest exercises with lighter weights, and by focusing on squeezing your chest. Or by simply flexing and forcing blood into the muscle. Try your best to feel your muscles contract at the peak of the movement. This is not about weights, it is about form and focusing on how these movements activate your muscles. From there, you can move into your main workout, but the initial pump might help you to connect your mind to your muscles more easily.

My personal favorite way to achieve this is through using an abduction method, which is essentially bringing your hands together. To do this, simply grab two 5-pound plates and place them in your palms. Push the two plates together using only your palms— do not use your fingers to hold the plates in place as this will activate the use of different muscles. Use only the force generated from the chest to push the plates together. Do this in a pressing motion and squeeze your chest when you push the plates together while extending your arms out. Repeating exercises such as this helps to get an initial pump on your chest and activate your pectoral muscles.

When working on your chest, it also helps to visualize what the muscles are doing as you work them. Let us look at how you would activate this connection when using the bench press. When your hands are getting closer to your chest, or on your descent, imagine your pecs being stretched out to the sides. When the weights are at chest level, hold your position for a moment and focus on your pecs being stretched out. Then, when you are ready to push up again, imagine squeezing your pecs together in the middle and pushing forward with them. Visualization is key here. In your mind's eye, you should see the inner muscles of your pecs stretching and contracting as you bench press.

Achieving the mind-to-muscle connection in the glutes tends to come more naturally to most people. However, there are still some tips and tricks we can use. One of the most important ones is to warm up and activate your glutes before you start working out. The use of bands can help a lot with this. One exercise you can do is banded bodyweight squats. Place the band just above your knees and stand with feet a little wider than shoulder-width, with your toes pointed slightly outwards in order to better target the glutes. In this stance, you are going to do about 20 squats (BlenderBottle Trainer Team, 2019). Be conscious of your glutes as you do this, doing the movements slowly and deliberately. Most importantly, squeeze your glutes as you get to the top of the movement at the end of each squat.

This will warm up your glutes, helping you to feel them. It will also get you into the headspace of controlled and deliberate movements, and allow you to focus solely on your glutes as you work them. It is important to maintain the mind-to-muscle connection you have established in that activation throughout the workout. Don't forget, one of the best ways to continue to feel your glutes is to really squeeze them at the top of every movement. For example, if you are doing weighted hip thrusts, you should stop at the top of every rep and squeeze your glutes when you are at full hip extension. Do not just get to the top and bring your hips back down again. You should go slowly through the movements and then stop at the top for at least a second or two. Then, you can slowly bring your hips back down again. This allows you to actually think about your glute muscles that you are trying to grow and allows your mind to connect to them.

Next, we will look at isolating your shoulders but more specifically your side and rear deltoids. In order to better target and isolate both your side delts and rear delts you are going to want to feel like you are pushing your elbows away from your body, not upwards, not backward but away from your body.

This is similar to isolating your back by focusing on the movement of your elbows but rather than pulling with them you are feeling as if you are pushing them outwards. The difference would be for rear delts your body would be closer to parallel with the ground and for side delts, your body would be closer to perpendicular with the ground. More than any other body part, in order to feel the work within your delts you will want to fully control and slow the movement of the weights as they descend down.

Having a solid mind to muscle connection for your biceps is something that seems to come naturally to people. But with a couple of tricks, you can increase the efficiency of your curls 10-fold. In order to do this, you will want to squeeze your pinky tighter than the rest of your hand. As you are standing with the weights at your side you will want your thumbs to be facing forward as if you were going to do a hammer curl then as you bring the weight up you will want to have supination of your hand so at the top of the curl your pinkies are pointing towards your ear. If you are doing curls with a bar try rather than having your wrists locked straight have them cocked back a little bit. This will give you a more isolated, harder flex on the bicep.

Lastly, we will look at achieving the connection with the muscles in our legs. Developing the mind-to-muscle connection when you are training your legs can be tricky too, but there are a few ways to make it easier. Legs are definitely one of the muscle groups that are easier to connect to through isolation movements rather than compound ones. Because of this, avoid lunges and opt instead to start with high-rep isolated movements such as leg curls and leg extensions. This will allow you to better focus on one muscle, for example, your hamstrings, rather than multiple muscles at once. Movements like leg curls and extensions also allow you to both stretch and squeeze your muscles, which helps to develop the connection.

When using the leg curl machine, set it to a lower weight than you would usually use. And just as you have done with the other exercises, take it slow. Make sure you are moving slowly and contracting and holding the muscles the whole time instead of swinging them. When you get to the top of the movement, contract and squeeze your hamstrings and hold the position for a second or two. Then slowly go back again. The key to these movements is time and contraction.

With all of these movements, it will just take time to find the positions in each rep where you feel them. Once you understand how to move in order to trigger the connection, it is just a matter of repeating that movement over and over again. Once you get into the habit, it will eventually become something that comes naturally. Using the mind-to-muscle connection in your workouts is essential for making progress. If you have been neglecting it so far in your fitness journey, it is undoubtedly why you are not seeing significant results.

CHAPTER 3: THE TRAINING STYLES YOU NEED TO KNOW

Now that we have established your diet and the mindset you need while you are working out, let us look at the different kinds of training styles that you can use to structure your workouts. If you are new to your fitness journey—even if you are in the middle of your journey—you might not have realized that there are different kinds of weight training. One of the main reasons that people don't see the changes they want is that they are not aware of the different styles of training. It might be that they are not training in the style that is suited for their goals, or maybe they are not using a combination of different styles that would get them the results that they want. We are going to make sure that you do not make that mistake.

There are a few different types of training that you can employ that benefit you in different ways. The ones we are going to look at are hypertrophy, strength training, endurance training, and speed and agility training. It is important that you know all of them, how they can help you, and how you can implement them into your workouts. Some of these will help you to build muscle, while some will make you stronger or make you able to work out for longer periods of time. All have their place in your routine, but you may find some more beneficial for your purposes than others. What's beneficial for you depends entirely on what you are trying to get out of your workouts. So let's dive into them!

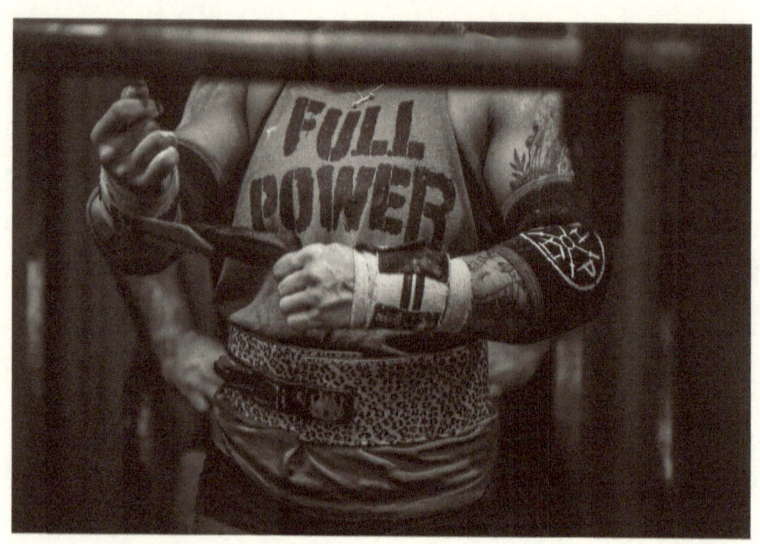

Hypertrophy

The ultimate muscle-building method is hypertrophy. Hypertrophy is defined as the "increase in muscular size when achieved through exercise" (Chertoff, 2019). Hypertrophy training helps to increase your muscle size and tone them. Of all the training styles we are going to look at, hypertrophy is the one that will help you to build a more muscular body than the other training styles. While you begin to slowly build your strength, you will be able to build the physique of your dreams. "The goal isn't to be able to lift 1000 pounds the goal is to look like you can" (Bmeade, 2021)

There are two different types of hypertrophy: myofibrillar and sarcoplasmic. Myofibrillar training grows the parts of your muscles that are responsible for contraction and tends to help with strength and speed. Sarcoplasmic training increases the storage of glycogen in your muscles, and this helps to give your body more sustained energy for endurance events, such as marathons.

To achieve hypertrophy in your muscles, you have to have both mechanical damage and metabolic fatigue. When you lift heavy, you do mechanical damage to your muscles. In order to fight against the resistance of the weights, the muscles responsible for contraction need to generate a certain amount of force. This causes structural damage to the protein in the muscles, and a repair response is stimulated in the body. When the muscle is repaired, it causes an increase in muscle size.

Metabolic fatigue is caused when your muscles use up their stores of energy. This energy is known as adenosine triphosphate, or ATP, and it is energy that helps your muscles to contract. When you lift, you are constantly contracting your muscles, so ATP depletes quickly. When this is depleted, the muscles will no longer be fueled for contractions and you won't be able to lift the weight properly. This is how you reach your max. When your ATP is depleted, this can also lead to muscle growth (Krzysztofik et al., 2019).

It is through both of these biological functions that you achieve hypertrophy in your muscles. However, hypertrophy-based workouts do not require you to hit failure with every exercise you do—in other words, stopping when you can no longer follow through with the rep without affecting your form. There just needs to be a significant amount of muscle tension, as well as metabolic stress.

Hypertrophy training is used mostly for aesthetic gains. It is often used by bodybuilders in order to look larger and more muscular. It is the training style for maximizing your muscle gains if that is what you are after. But this kind of training can also be beneficial from a health standpoint. Increasing your muscle mass contributes to a decrease in the risk of health concerns, such as cardiovascular disease and type 2 diabetes in middle-aged and older adults (Krzysztofik et al., 2019).

There are many factors that influence the effectiveness of a hypertrophy workout, most notably the volume and intensity. The routine recommended by the American College of Sports Medicine (ACSM) for a novice is to do between 1–3 sets of each exercise, with between 8–12 reps in each set (American College of Sports Medicine, 2009).

When choosing the weight for your exercise, it is important to lift weight that is challenging, but also one with which you are able to maintain your form. The weight you are lifting during this kind of training is not the most important thing, rather it is the wearing out of your muscles through repetition and intensity. While weights can help with this, they should not be so heavy that you cannot complete your 8-12 reps, or so heavy that you have to allow for long pauses in between sets to catch your breath.

It is also helpful to increase the weights you are lifting gradually. Do not aim to increase weight with every workout, for example, but maybe aim to go up in weight every week or two in your various exercises. For this style of training, you would do a reps-and-rest cycle when you train. You should allow for 60–90 seconds rest between sets. This helps to fatigue the muscles and achieve hypertrophy.

Your range of motion during your reps is also important during hypertrophy training. You need to push your muscles by achieving the full range with every rep. This does not mean that you lock out on every rep. You want to keep the tension on your muscles the entire time not your joints That is also why using a weight you can control is essential. You can also cause progressive overloading by increasing your range of motion over time, instead of upping your weight. For example, you can focus on making sure your form and control over the weight you are using is spot on and you can control the weight easier each time you use them.

Lastly, one of the keys to continually fatiguing your muscles is by changing up the way you are working them. You should vary the exercises you do in each workout, as it can help to fire up different muscles and fibers. Changing what you do every couple of weeks is also helpful as it fatigues a wide range of different muscles, allowing you to see the best and most even results.

Strength Training

While hypertrophy training helps you to build the ideal physique and get you stronger, it will not necessarily help you to get stronger like strength training will. Building strength is very different from building mass. If your goal is to constantly hit new personal bests, strength training is where you will find yourself meeting those kinds of goals. Unlike hypertrophy training, strength training aims for increased ability, rather than an increase in muscle mass. While you will still create muscle mass through strength training, that is not the goal. The goal is to get strong. Bodybuilders do hypertrophy training in order to look good, but athletes such as strongmen and strongwomen will do strength training that will prepare them to tackle the insanely heavy loads that they lift in their competitions. Strength training focuses on fewer reps and longer rest periods than hypertrophy training; your max number of reps will be 6 instead of 12.

You might consider strength training if you are looking to consistently obtain new PRs, or personal records. You can also use this method of training if your goal is to compete in lifting contests. If you just want to become stronger and more capable, and if you want your goals to be based on what you can do rather than how you look, strength training is the way to achieve that. Many people find this far more motivating, as they can see the amount of weight they are able to lift steadily increase as they train. Furthermore, strength training has several health benefits. For one, it helps to strengthen your bones, as it can increase bone density and reduce the risk of developing osteoporosis.

While strength training will not increase your muscle mass to the same extent as hypertrophy training, it will help you to lose fat (diet depending) and develop and maintain lean muscle. It increases your metabolism and helps you to lose weight. Developing lean muscle and becoming functionally stronger will also improve your everyday quality of life (Mayoclinic, 2019). When you build your skeletal muscle through consistent strength training, you improve your ability to complete everyday activities, you improve your balance, and a strong body can help you to age gracefully with fewer medical complications. Loss of skeletal muscle as we age can also lead to a slowed-down metabolic rate, which is a factor that contributes to weight gain and obesity (Thomas & Burns, 2019).

So let's look at how to use strength training in your weekly fitness routine. The focus in strength training is how much weight you can lift, and you should maximize your weight for the workout to be effective. The recommended number of reps for strength training is between 3-6 reps for each set. In general, the lower the rep range, the more your strength will increase. If you can do more than 6 reps, then your weight is too light, and your workout won't succeed in building your strength. But if you cannot complete at least 3 reps, then your weight is too heavy to achieve any results. Finding this balance is key for strength training.

You should also be testing the limits of what you can lift—it is only through continually pushing yourself that you will get stronger. If you find yourself getting through your workout easily, do not increase your reps, increase your weights. Weights are where you are going to get your strength. There are certain bodyweight exercises that will also help, such as push-ups and pullups, but you need to supplement your workouts with some form of resistance to feel the full effects, either in the form of weights or resistance bands.

Another thing to remember when it comes to strength training is the importance of rest, both in between your sets and in between your workouts. In between your sets, you should rest for at least a few minutes. If you do not, you will not be able to maintain the strength to lift heavily throughout your workout. For example, let us say for your first set you can squat 150 lbs. for six reps. If you try to do your second set after less than a minute of rest, you will undoubtedly be unable to repeat the set with that weight— or if you can, it means that your weights are too light. If your weights are heavy enough, you should need at least a few minutes of rest between sets to achieve another set of 6 at 150 lbs. You can wait for up to 5–10 minutes between sets if that's the time it takes for you to recover (Aceto, 2003). The more time you allow between sets, the more weight you will be able to lift. And high weight is key to developing strength. This is one of the main differences between hypertrophy and strength training. You are aiming to fatigue your muscles, but just over a longer period and with heavier weights.

Just as rest between sets is important, allowing yourself a significant number of rest days in your week is also important. Allowing a few rest days a week allows your muscles to recover, meaning that you will be refreshed when coming back for your next training day. If you do not allow for rest days, your muscles will be constantly fatigued, and you will be unable to keep lifting heavy weights consistently. Because you are using heavier weights with strength training, rest days are especially important because allowing your muscles time to recover properly helps to prevent injury. For strength training, it is recommended you take at least two rest days per week to see significant results. Allowing yourself time to warm up before strength training is also very important. As previously mentioned, the lifting of heavy weights can lead to injury if you are not careful and mindful of proper form (Mayoclinic, 2019). Warming up with stretching and 10 minutes of aerobic exercise can help to warm up your muscles and prevent injury.

A deload week from time to time will help you out as well. Basically, just take the movements that you were doing for 3-6 reps and try to do a moderate weight for 20-25 reps. It will give your joints and tendons a break and allow you to perfect your form and still get the blood moving around your body with a good pump.

Endurance Training

The third style of training that you can focus on is endurance training. Endurance training enables your muscles to perform things repeatedly and for extended periods of time. It will not make an obvious aesthetic difference in your muscles like hypertrophy, nor will it make you stronger as strength training does. Rather, including endurance training in your workout allows you to work out for longer periods, to perform reps repeatedly, and helps to prevent injury. Your endurance is made up of two components—your cardiovascular endurance and your muscular endurance. Cardiovascular endurance is the ability of your heart and lungs to supply your body with oxygen when under stress. Muscular endurance is the ability of your muscles to work for long periods of time without getting fatigued (Yetman, 2020). In order to improve your cardiovascular endurance, you should look at exercises such as running, walking, jump rope, or swimming. These can supplement your weightlifting, and will also help you to work on your muscular endurance. Working on your muscular endurance requires weightlifting endurance training.

Endurance training is usually helpful as support for the other types of training that you may do. Some people focus on their muscular endurance in order to aid in their strength or hypertrophy training. If their muscles can be worked for longer, they can get a more effective workout. Other people do both cardiovascular and muscular endurance to aid in other physical activities that they do. For example, those who run marathons and engage in sports such as cycling, running, and rock climbing use endurance training to improve their performance in those areas. Ex-athletes also tend to do endurance training. This allows them to maintain their muscle mass and strength without putting the same strain on their body that they did when they were competing.

Endurance training is beneficial for everyone, from professional athletes to marathon runners to everyday recreational athletes. It allows you to train longer and harder when doing the other different styles of training, therefore it improves your performance. It is also easier on your body and helps with your recovery. Endurance is also healthy for your heart, your circulatory system, and lungs. It is a type of maintenance: exercises that will still work you but are not always as intense or taxing on your body. This type of training can make everyday life easier; if you struggle to breathe once you get up a flight of stairs, endurance training is something you should look into.

In terms of developing muscle and strength, endurance training helps to increase existing muscle strength and size, however, it will not develop muscle if it is not already there. Endurance training is a good way to deload from your normal weightlifting strain. It allows you to give your muscles a bit of a rest, while still maintaining the mass and strength in your muscles. It allows you to perform the same exercises, but with less intensity.

Endurance training is all about using light weights (or even bodyweight) and focusing on repetition. The minimum amount of reps you should be doing in any set is 15, but you can go all the way up to 40 reps per exercise. If you cannot make it to at least 15 reps with ease, you should lower your weights. However, if you are not experiencing any strain at all after 40 or so reps, you need to up the weight. Even a slight increase of 2 lbs. will make a significant difference when doing endurance training because you are doing so many reps. It is not about using your maximum amount of strength; you should only be using about 50% of your maximum power. In between sets, you should only rest for about 20 seconds.

One of the common ways to do endurance training is by doing circuits. Training circuits consist of three or more exercises completed in a routine one after the other, either based on number of reps or on a time limit. You then rest for two minutes and start the circuit again. Also, endurance training does not necessarily need to be split into different muscle groups. You can work the full body or multiple muscle groups in one endurance training session. Or you can split it how you would your strength or hypertrophy training workouts, and simply cut back the weights and rest time, and bump up the reps.

There are a number of things you should do when endurance training. Firstly, it is important to stay hydrated. While this is true for any exercise, it is especially true for endurance training because you are pushing for muscle fatigue. Failing to stay hydrated can lead to muscle cramps and can hinder your performance. It can cause your muscles to grow fatigued too quickly, as a lack of water can deplete your level of electrolytes (Grinnell, 2019). It is also important to warm up dynamically. When you stretch, make sure they are dynamic stretches or bodyweight drills. For example, you can do squats, lunges, and jumping jacks. Because endurance training is fast paced, it is important to warm up your muscles in preparation for the work they need to do.

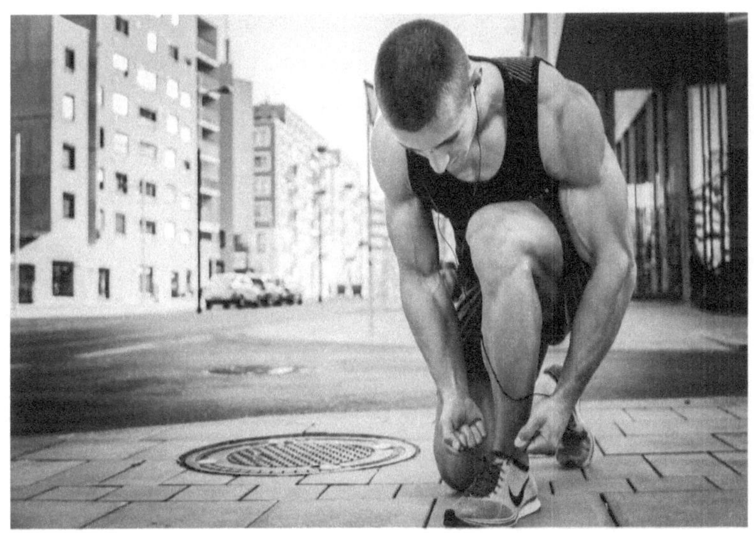

Speed and Agility Training

The last style of training that you need to know is speed and agility training. This type of training will not necessarily increase your muscle mass, strength, or endurance, but it will help to make you a more well-rounded athlete. Many weightlifters do not tend to focus on speed and agility training, as they do not think it is relevant to what they are trying to achieve. If you are aiming to build your strength, and are focusing on slow and deliberate movements, why would you worry about training for speed or agility? However, training your speed and agility is essential for balance and coordination, which will ultimately give you greater control over your body and aid your weightlifting and other training.

One of the most common types of training for speed is performing simple speed drills, most of which include repetitive sprinting, high kicks, and running up and down stairs or bleachers. You set up a certain distance and time yourself and aim to do a certain number of laps within that space of time. Each time, you should try to up the number of laps you can do within the time limit. This training can also include doing dot drills, high-knee drills, or lateral drills. Another type is resisted speed training. This is when you perform the same speed drills but with added resistance. For example, many football and rugby players will do sprinting drills while dragging a sled that is attached to their center mass, around their waist. However, it is important that the added resistance is not training your strength instead of your speed. If the weight is too heavy, you will struggle to move because you are too weighed down. You will then muscle your way through the drill, and you will be improving your strength instead of your speed. However, if you use a lower weight, it will add resistance but still allow you to run in your natural running rhythm (Richey, 2018).

There is also assistance training, whereby you use some type of aid to help yourself to move faster than you could on your own. This can be done by running downhill or using bungee cords. Both of those help to increase speed when practiced over time.

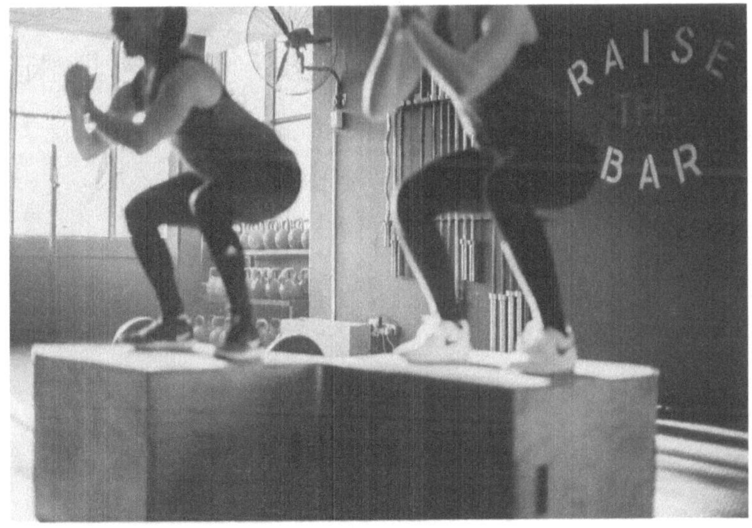

The best way to train for speed and agility is undoubtedly plyometric training. Plyometric exercises are aerobic exercises that increase your endurance, your speed, and your agility. Unlike strength training, which focuses on slow, long, and deliberate movements, plyometric training is all about moving through the exercise quickly and with grace. Plyometric training helps to build your speed and agility because these movements cause our brains to activate multiple muscle fibers at once, and almost instantaneously. Doing this type of exercise increases the efficiency of our muscle contractions, and your body becomes quicker and more agile the more you do it.

The main idea behind plyometrics is based upon making the stretch-shortening cycle (SSC) happen as quickly as possible. This is the process your muscles go through when you move dynamically. The muscle is stretched first when you make a dynamic movement, which is also known as an eccentric movement. The muscle then contracts or makes a concentric movement. For example, when you dip down to do a tuck jump, your center of mass is lowered quickly, which causes your muscles to stretch. You will then contract your leg muscles—your quads and your hamstrings—to push you into the air for the tuck jump. These two movements together are known as the SSC, and together they cause a more powerful contraction than what was caused by a concentric movement alone (Imbo, 2014). By making the SSC happen as quickly as possible, your movement will become quicker. Plyometric training aims to do just that.

Plyometric training also used to be known as 'jump training' because it involves a series of movements dependent on jumping. You can incorporate a box and do box jumps or use steps to do stairway hops. You can also involve jumping in many of your regular movements—for example, you can do jump squats, jump lunges, or jumping lateral lunges. You can also do movements such as burpees and tuck jumps.

Speed and agility training has a number of benefits. These exercises help to prevent injuries because they increase the strength of the tendons. Plyometrics especially aid in improving the elasticity of your tendons because it places stress on them in a controlled setting. This is especially beneficial for weightlifting. Weightlifting places a large amount of strain on your tendons and requires a huge burst of power from your muscles in a short space of time. Therefore, protecting your tendons and making them stronger is essential.

Plyometric training also helps to boost the effectiveness of your neuromuscular system. As previously mentioned, strength and agility training helps to shorten the process of your muscle stretching and contracting, the SCC. When this happens, a signal is sent to your muscles from your brain via the neuromuscular system. The quicker this transmission happens, the faster you can contract and stretch your muscles. Therefore, the more you do this style of training, the quicker and more effective your neuromuscular system becomes and the faster you can move. This is beneficial for any other form of activity that you do.

It has also been found that incorporating speed and agility training can help lifters improve their power output and decrease the time it takes for them to reach maximum force (Imbo, 2014). While speed and agility training isn't essential, it will give an edge to the rest of your workouts that you would be foolish not to want. Lastly, most of these exercises require very little equipment or can be done outside the gym. A change of scenery can create some nice, welcome variety in your weekly workout routine.

One of the biggest mistakes people make is not having an aim for their training, and unintentionally using a mix of all of these styles in their workouts without understanding how different rep ranges and rest periods affect them. For example, if you have been going to the gym for years looking to build muscle, and you have been doing 6 reps with high weights for most exercises, you are not going to see the results that you want because you were unintentionally doing strength training instead of hypertrophy.

Most people will benefit from using a mix of these styles of training. If you are looking to improve your fitness and develop a muscular or lean physique, you might find yourself including different aspects of each of the training styles in your routine. You can focus some days on strength, some on hypertrophy, a few on endurance, and a few on speed and agility training. Or maybe you'll find that you only want to use one or two of these training styles in your routine because you don't need the other ones. You can split these training styles up by days, or even spend months alternating, depending on what you are trying to build. It depends entirely on what your goals are. By understanding all of these styles and what they will do for you, you will be better informed to know how you need to train to reach the goals that you have set for yourself.

CHAPTER 4: HOW TO FIND YOUR IDEAL CARDIO

If your main focus is building muscle, cardio can often be neglected in favor of lifting weights and other strength exercises. A lot of people simply do not enjoy cardio or find it hard to see why it is so important. But cardio is crucial for reaching your goals for many reasons. It helps to burn fat, which is important for achieving a lean physique and being able to see the muscles gained from weightlifting. It will also keep you healthy in the long term. Cardio helps to prevent the many health issues that come with aging, such as heart disease, cholesterol and blood pressure problems, as well as a variety of other cardiovascular conditions. In order to achieve your fitness goals, cardio needs to be an essential component of your weekly workout routine. Together with strength training, cardio exercises will help you to develop bone density, lose fat, and get strong.

So, what is cardio? Cardio is an aerobic exercise, and aerobic basically means "with oxygen." Cardio itself is short for cardiovascular, as any form of cardio engages your cardiovascular system.

These kinds of exercises should give you the feeling of your heart racing, your blood pumping, and a shortness of breath.

Cardio is any exercise where you are moving. It is the process of repeatedly moving the larger muscles that make up your body, such as the ones in your legs, your arms, and your hips (Lavie et al., 2015).

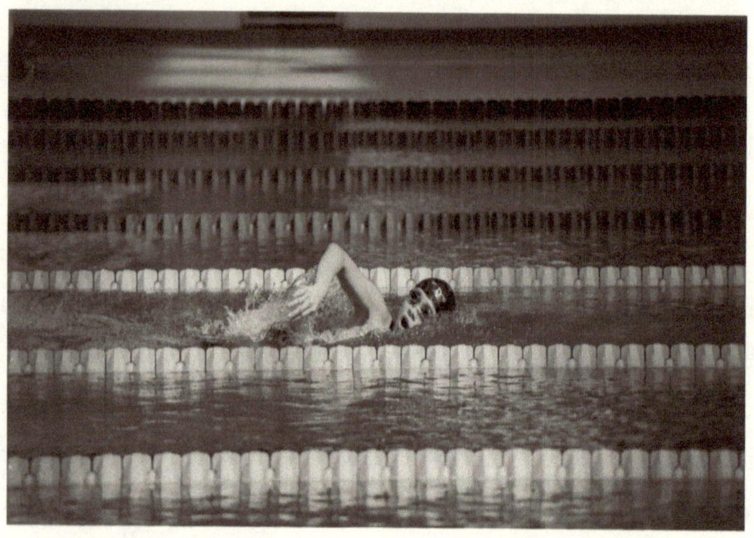

The most common forms of cardio are activities like running, walking, and swimming, however, they are not the only ones. Dancing can be cardio. So can doing high-intensity interval training (HIIT), or kickboxing classes, or hiking. Many people tend to dread cardio because they have a limited view of what they have to do for cardio. You do not have to spend an hour every day running on the treadmill or devote large chunks of your week to cycling or swimming. If you enjoy that kind of movement, go for it! But there are dozens of different cardio exercises that you can incorporate into your routine. They all have different functions, and you can therefore pick and choose depending on what you need and what you enjoy doing most. After all, you want your workouts to be a sustainable part of your lifestyle, and it's much easier to sustain activities you enjoy!

It's also important to understand how cardio contributes to the rest of your fitness routine. There are different benefits depending on when you chose to incorporate cardio into your routine. We will explore that, as well as a few different options for cardio that can improve your life and fitness in several different ways.

There is some debate among fitness experts concerning the best time to do cardio, however, when you choose to do it depends entirely on your goals. People tend to disagree about the benefits of doing cardio before your weightlifting workout versus after your workout, for example, and we will explore that issue later.

There is also the question of fasted cardio. Fasted cardio involves doing aerobic exercise, or raising your heart rate, without eating something beforehand. Ideally, you should have a completely empty stomach, and it is therefore recommended that you do fasted cardio first thing in the morning before eating breakfast. While you may think that you have an empty stomach by 4 p.m. if you ate lunch at 1 p.m. with no snacks in between, that is not necessarily true. Your stomach is probably still digesting your lunch. The ideal time to do fasted cardio is when your insulin level is at baseline and your body isn't digesting or absorbing nutrients. Depending on what you ate (the volume, the macronutrients, and the calories) and your individual, unique body, it can take anywhere from 3 to 6 hours after you have eaten to get to this 'fasted' state (Schinetsky, 2019). Since it is almost impossible to pinpoint when you would reach this state after a meal, it is easier to just do cardio in the morning on an empty stomach.

Fasted cardio is highly effective for weight loss. One of the best ways to achieve this is to walk on a treadmill at a speed of around 2.8 to 3.0 miles per hour on a high incline. You can also go for a fast walk outside. Fasted cardio should be low intensity, the kind where you are not completely out of breath and are still able to hold a conversation while exercising.

However, it's best to avoid intense activity on an empty stomach. It can be dangerous to do high-intensity workouts without eating first, as you are more likely to feel weak and tired and you are more prone to injury. Furthermore, your body might become so desperate for energy that it will start breaking down your muscle tissue as well as your fat tissue. This is because your muscle contains glycogen and stores glucose, and it will use that to fuel your muscles if you are putting them under intense strain (Kassel, 2019). Therefore, you could lose muscle mass by doing more intense workouts while fasting. This is one of the few times where it is better to stick to activities which are slow and steady.

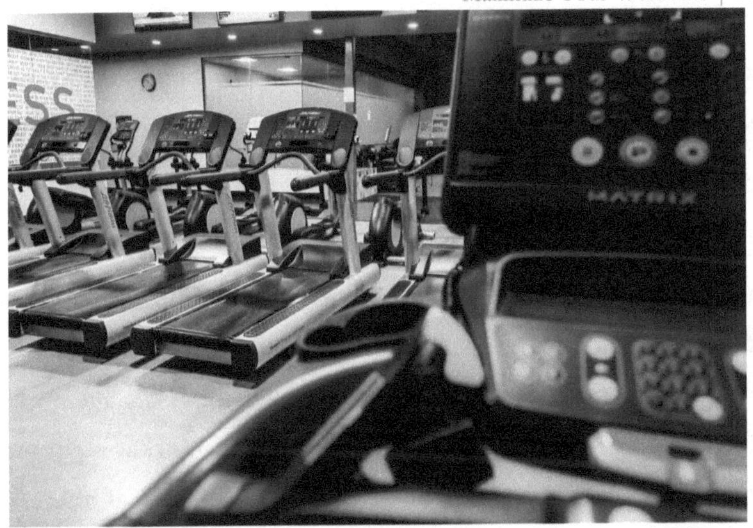

The main benefit of fasted cardio is that it burns fat. Studies have shown that fasted cardio burns considerably more fat than doing the same level of activity when you have a full stomach because it induces higher fat oxidation (Schinetsky, 2019). This is because your body will always burn the nutrients that are readily available first. Therefore, if you have just eaten, your body will burn that food in order to get energy. Once those calories have been burned, it will then begin burning up your body fat, which serves as energy stores, in order to keep the body moving. However, if you have nothing in your stomach, your body will resort to burning up your fat. Doing this consistently trains your body to burn up fat for energy, and you will see your body fat declining rapidly in no time.

Fasted cardio also helps to lose stubborn fat. Everyone has some level of fat that they cannot get rid of no matter how hard they try. Maybe you have always had a stomach pouch, or maybe your thighs are the last part of your body to slim down.

Maybe no matter what you do, you can't budge past a certain number on the scale. The reason that some body fat is more stubborn is dependent on the amount of blood flow it receives, as well as the ratio of alpha to beta cells in those areas.

Fat cells have two types of receptors—alpha and beta receptors. Alpha receptors reduce fat burning, while beta receptors encourage fat burning. Therefore, the more alpha receptors a fat cell has, the more it resists releasing its stored fatty acids to be burned up for energy. This is what stubborn fat is generally made up of. This is made worse if there is limited blood flow to that area (Schinetsky, 2019). Fasted cardio tends to help with stubborn fat because it increases blood flow, particularly to the abdomen, which is where most people experience stubborn fat that they cannot lose. Increased blood flow means the tissue is more likely to release its stored fatty acid to be used up.

The other option for when to incorporate cardio is after your workout. There are a number of benefits to this too. Doing cardio after you lift is often better than doing it before because it prevents you from feeling fatigued for your weightlifting. Cardio is tiring, both for your muscles and your mind. Studies have shown that doing cardio depletes your muscular endurance, as well as your focus and energy. You need all of these things to lift. Lifting is hard and requires you to have all your physical and mental reserves to do it, otherwise, you will start to sacrifice proper form and technique due to fatigue. This could lead to injury, as well as prevent you from progressing at the rate that you should because your sessions are never optimal (Boly, 2021).

There are several benefits associated with doing cardio after you have done a strength workout. Your heart rate will already be up from your workout, so you will start burning fat immediately instead of having to work up to it. Doing cardio after you work out also primes your body to build more muscle and allows you to lift heavier weights because of how the enzymes and energy in your body respond to cardio after lifting weights versus the other way around (Boly, 2021). When doing cardio after your workout, you have a few more options than you do when you are doing fasted cardio because your body is fueled. You can still do the brisk walk mentioned earlier for fasted cardio, however, you can also do more high-intensity forms of movements, such as sprints and high-intensity interval training. You can also use cardio machines, such as the elliptical or the StairMaster and amp up the intensity as high as you want.

Both fasted cardio and post-workout cardio will help you to burn fat, which is the most common goal of cardio. There is little difference in the results that come from fasted cardio versus post workout cardio. What you choose to do will be dependent on what type of cardio you enjoy as well as what fits more comfortably in your schedule.

Fasted cardio is beneficial for fat loss because it targets your stored fat. Many people prefer to do fasted cardio because they can get it out of the way early in the day, and they don't have to worry about finding another time of the day to fit it in.

On the other hand, you might not be a morning person. Or you might already have to start your day very early in the morning so waking up even earlier to get your cardio in may be too much of a struggle. Or maybe you just want to get your entire workout for the day done at once, and you would rather just do your cardio after your lifting routine because you're already at the gym, your heart rate is already up, and therefore you start burning fat immediately. It will be easier to stick to cardio if it fits into your routine, especially if you are not the kind of person who is overly excited by the prospect of doing cardio. With post-workout cardio, you also have more options available to you, and it might therefore be easier for you to maintain a cardio routine if you enjoy some variety in the types of activities you do. At the end of the day, when you do cardio is a personal choice. Either of these methods will help you to achieve your goal, you just need to find what works best for you.

How much cardio you need to do each week is also dependent on your goals. If you are trying to lose weight and gain lean muscle, you should aim to do more cardio, while if you are trying to bulk up and gain only muscle, you should do a little bit less. In general, you should incorporate cardio between 2–4 times per week, for anywhere from 30 minutes to an hour. If you are trying to add bulk, aim to do 2 days of cardio a week for 30–40 minutes each time. If you are looking to lose fat, aim to do 4 days a week, doing an hour of cardio for 2 of those days and 30 minutes for the other 2 days. You need to find what works for you and your goals.

Now that we have looked at the different ways to schedule your cardio, let us look at the differences between high-intensity cardio training, also known as HIIT, and low-intensity training.

A common misconception is that cardio is only effective if it is intense, if your heart is racing and you are dripping with sweat after 10 minutes. However, low-intensity cardio is just as effective and has different benefits for your body than high-intensity cardio does. One of the main differences is the length of time, and obviously, the level of intensity.

Low-intensity cardio can take anywhere from 30 minutes to an hour, and you should be exercising at a low enough level that you could hold a conversation for the duration of your movement. High-intensity cardio, on the other hand, is usually never longer than 20 minutes. You should be breathless the whole time and ready to collapse at the end of it. A few examples of HIIT exercises are sprints, jumping rope, running stairs, and HIIT circuit cardio training. Some examples of the exercises you would do in HIIT cardio circuits would be burpees, jumping jacks, or jump squats.

HIIT is an interval workout, so that means short bursts of very high energy, intense movements followed by brief moments of rest or low-intensity activity. For example, you could have 40 seconds of jumping jacks, followed by 10 seconds of jogging on the spot. And then repeat. Next, you could do 40 seconds of burpees and 10 seconds of rest. And then repeat. Your heart rate should be between 120 and 150 beats per minute the entire time (depending on your age; optimal heart rate for fat burning is lower for people over 50 years of age).

There are a number of benefits from doing high-intensity cardio. Chiefly, it burns a lot of calories in a short amount of time, which can help you to lose fat. It is estimated that HIIT burns 25-30% more calories than any other form of exercise. A lot of this happens after you do the routine, as your metabolic rate is higher for hours afterward. HIIT increases your metabolism after exercise more than most other forms of exercise, even jogging and weightlifting. It helps to build muscle too. Although HIIT is cardio focused, you are also powering the movements through muscle, mainly those in your legs and glutes. Therefore, you might see muscle growth in those areas. It can also reduce blood sugar, blood pressure, and cholesterol (Tinsley, 2017).

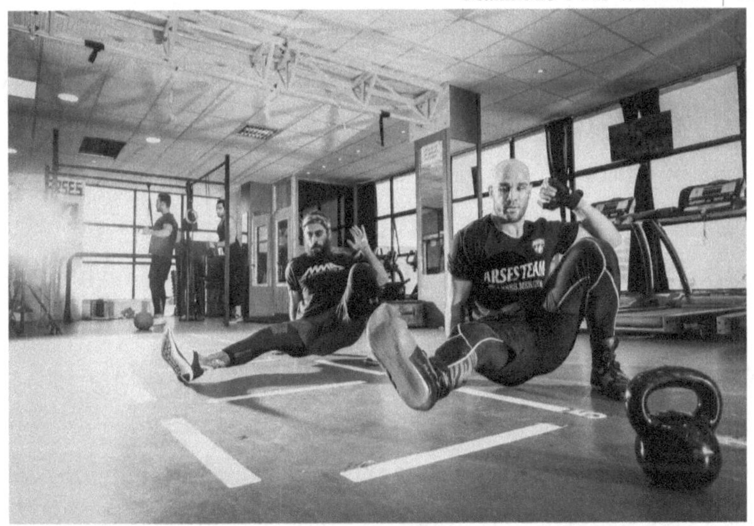

A low-intensity cardio workout will look very different. You can do low-intensity cardio for up to an hour, and your heart rate should be between 110–130, or about 60–70% of your maximum heart rate, for the duration of the workout. Just as with the morning walks mentioned in our discussion on fasted cardio, you should be able to hold a conversation the entire time you're performing low-intensity cardio. You should be moving at a consistent and steady pace, one that you can maintain for the duration of your workout. The best form of low-intensity cardio was already mentioned under fasted cardio—putting the treadmill on an incline and walking briskly. You can also do this by walking outside, but try to find areas with a lot of hills. Another great activity is hiking, but make sure the trails you choose are not too strenuous or rocky.

Many people prefer low-intensity cardio training over high-intensity training because it still burns a fair amount of calories and it does so without putting the same amount of strain on your body. Because high-intensity requires such dynamic and intense movement, people who do it often are more prone to injury than those who stick to low-intensity. People who have problems with their joints—their wrists, ankles, and knees, for example—will struggle to do high-intensity routines a few times a week. And because HIIT is also more draining on your energy, you may find that low-intensity exercises still leave you with the energy to go about the rest of your day— without aching muscles.

Furthermore, although HIIT burns more calories, it has been proven that low-intensity exercise tends to burn more fat. While doing HIIT, your body does burn fat, but will also break down and use some of the energy stored in your muscles for fuel. However, during low-intensity, your body is more likely to just burn stored fat. Therefore, low intensity is better for fat loss.

It is often a good idea to mix up both types of cardio into your workout routine, as they both are beneficial for different reasons. Some days you might only have time for HIIT because it takes far less time than low-intensity workouts, and other days your muscles might be sore from lifting and so you'd rather opt for a low-intensity cardio routine. How you decide to split your workouts between the types of cardio is purely up to you.

You will see the benefits of cardio not only in your other workouts, but in your life in general. Cardio has huge benefits for your heart and overall cardiovascular health. It leads to decreases in your resting heart rate, as well as your blood pressure, which means your heart does not have to work unnecessarily hard all the time. This can also help prevent heart disease as you age.

Cardio is beneficial for other parts of your body too, particularly your brain and your joints. It increases blood flow to the brain, and this is beneficial for preventing conditions such as dementia and stroke. It also helps in general brain functioning. You will find yourself more alert and attentive in your day-to-day life if you engage in regular cardio exercise (Cleveland Clinic, 2016). As previously mentioned, cardio also boosts your metabolism, burns a high number of calories, and burns off fat. If you are looking to lose weight or become more lean, cardio will be an essential part of your journey.

The increase in circulation that cardio causes have other benefits outside of your heart and organ health. The increased circulation leads to clear, healthy skin, and also plays a significant role in keeping your muscles supplied with oxygen. When your muscles are better supplied with oxygen, they are able to work harder. Over time, cardio also helps your muscles get used to an increased workload. Therefore, doing cardio greatly assists your weightlifting training and makes everyday tasks easier, as well.

Lastly, one of the greatest benefits of cardio is a boost in your mood and energy. Just think about how good you feel after a good workout! That is because exercising releases chemicals that make you happy. Doing cardio regularly releases a range of stress fighting endorphins, such as dopamine and serotonin. These hormones help to boost your mood from day to day and equip you to better handle stress. Regular cardio also releases endorphins throughout the day that give you significant amounts of lasting energy. Regular cardio also helps you to sleep better—both by helping you to fall asleep and achieve deep and consistent sleep.

Cardio is often viewed as the ugly stepchild of fitness, particularly by weightlifters and gym rats. It is something people tend to neglect when they are aiming to build muscle, or when most of their workout routine involves weightlifting. However, you will never reach your peak if you are not implementing cardio, even if it is only a few days a week.

If you have never incorporated cardio into your routine before, start small. Find a type of cardio that you enjoy and then promise to do it at least once a week. After a few weeks of this, bump it up to twice a week. And so forth. Try out different types of cardio and see what suits you. You will find a way to fit it in that suits your goals, your lifestyle, and your motivation. The health benefits are endless, and it is the foundation upon which you need to build the rest of your workout routine. Incorporating cardio into your week will not only allow you to see improvements in other areas of your fitness, but it will also improve your everyday quality of life.

If you feel healthy, fit, and energized all the time, it is easier to devote time to your fitness and health. That is why cardio is so important.

CHAPTER 5: BUILDING YOUR OWN WORKOUT ROUTINE

One of the biggest struggles that people new to the gym experience is what, exactly, to do. It can be overwhelming and terrifying to walk into the weight section of the gym, surrounded by muscular people that look like they're been working out since the day they climbed out of their crib. This can be even more intimidating if you do not know enough about what you are doing to even create a solid workout routine.

If you are an intermediate lifter, you might find that the workout routines you are currently using are starting to feel a bit old. Maybe you no longer feel the same burn in your muscles, or maybe you are just getting bored with the way things are right now. Your workouts should excite you; they should be something that you look forward to.

Or maybe, the routine you follow simply has not given you the results that you want. Learning to build a new kind of routine could be exactly the thing you need to get excited about working out and could help you reach the physique and level of strength that you have always wanted.

One of the greatest assets you will learn from this book is how to build your own workout routine, one that will continually challenge you and allow you to see progress. Once you have the basics, you will find yourself easily able to switch up the routine now and then and find new ways of doing things. This is an invaluable skill for anyone aiming for a fitness-based lifestyle. However, it is also something that you will find easier to do as you go along. The more time you spend deliberating about how to split your workouts and planning them out, the more practice you have, and so the better you become at it. But I am going to give you the foundation.

First and foremost, we need to talk about warming up. Warming up is an essential part of every workout you do and should never be skipped. It might be tempting to jump straight into your routine if you're rushed, or low on time. This is a huge mistake. You are setting yourself up for injury if you are not allowing your body to warm up. Muscles and tendons that have not been stretched out and warmed up are far more prone to injury than those that are. Furthermore, stretching out and warming up your muscles allows them to recover more quickly because it increases blood flow around the body. This means that your recovery periods will be shorter and more effective, and you will progress faster. It will also help with muscles soreness, so you won't have to spend the day after leg day hobbling around quite as much.

Bottom line: your workouts will be less effective if you do not warm up first. Warm-ups make you more flexible, allowing for a greater range of motion. A greater range of motion allows you to work harder, as you get deeper into each movement. It allows you to fully work your muscles (Cronkleton, 2012).

The first part of your warm-up should be stretching. You should allow a few moments to allow your muscles to stretch out. You should also focus on stretching out the parts of your body that you are going to work on. A warm-up can incorporate both stationary and moving or fluid stretches—you can do a sort of flow through all the different poses.

The next part of your warm-up should be dynamic. Doing a dynamic warm-up is important for several reasons. It brings the body temperature up, which increases blood flow and oxygen to the muscles, helping to prepare it for what it is about to do. Dynamic warm-ups are often a low-intensity version of the workout you are actually about to do. For example, if you were warming up for leg day, you would do squats, lunges, and deadlifts. These should be slow and deliberate movements, where you are focusing on moving your muscles more than working them. You can do this using body weights or very light weights.

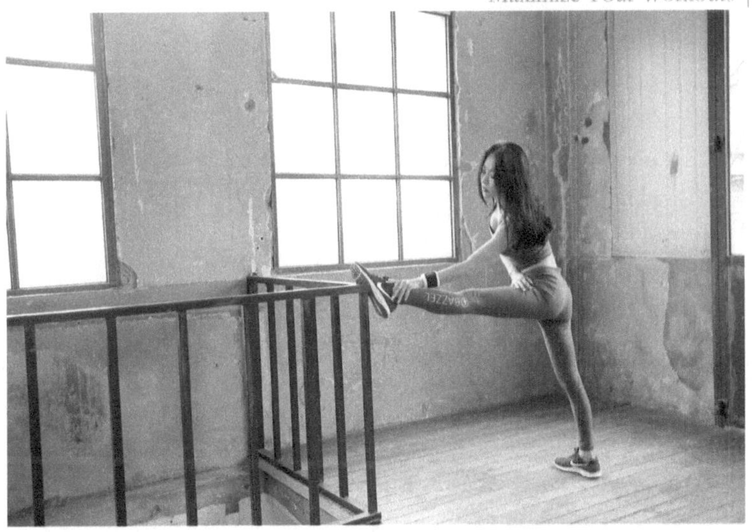

One of the first questions many people have when they start working out is how they should split up their workout. It's natural to feel overwhelmed with all the different options. How many days a week do I work out? How many rest days? Should I split the muscles in large groups, or do many days targeting individual muscles?

With so much uncertainty and so many options, one of the mistakes people make is to look up a professional weightlifter and just adopt their workout. I can understand the thinking: if I want to look like them, I'll train like them! However, they look and train like they do because they are professionals, and they have spent years building up their workout routine and their body. As a beginner, you should not follow a professional's routine, you should start off slowly. It is important to get your muscles used to the movement, and it is important to give your body time to build itself slowly and steadily. Without the foundation, you will never see the progress you want and may quit out of frustration.

When you are starting out, your focus should be on achieving the correct form and mastering your muscular coordination (Aceto, 2003). Both are required for continual growth. A beginner might be able to perfect their form, but if their muscle coordination is lacking, they will not be able to execute the movement when they start working with heavier weights.

You should also use this period of your training to master your mind-to-muscle connection. Because you are training with lower weights and with less intensity than you will later on, it is the ideal time to fully focus on feeling your muscles when you work out. As you progressively add more weights, it becomes harder to focus on the muscle you are working, as you are only able to focus on pushing the weight and finishing the rep. But if you have already mastered your mind-to-muscle connection as a beginner, you will naturally focus on feeling your muscle because you have made it a habit. The more time you give yourself in the beginning to solidify your base, the better you will progress in the future. You will be able to build the body and strength you have always wanted, it just takes time.

So, what is the ideal workout split for beginners? When you start, you should be aiming to train 3 days a week. For each of the three workouts, you will focus on two different body parts. For those two body parts, you will perform two exercises each in the very beginning then up that up to 3 after a couple weeks. This allows you to have a rest day in between each workout.

So, you would work out one day, take off the next, workout the day after that, and so on. This allows your body to get used to the movements and the weights, without overloading it. Remember: The rest days are an important part of this schedule.

There are two different ways to split the muscle groups you would work in each day. The first option is as follows: Monday, you train your back and triceps; Wednesday, you train your legs and your shoulders; and Friday, you train your chest and your biceps.

The second option is to split the workouts for your upper body into a push and pull day, and then also do a leg day. Let's say, for example, you decided to do a pull workout on Monday. This would essentially mean that you are training your back and your biceps—all the muscles you use to pull the weights up or towards you. On Wednesday, you would do a push workout, so you would be working any muscle that requires you to push something—any exercise where you would be pushing the weights away from you in any direction such as chest, triceps and shoulders. Then on Friday, you would train legs. This is a good way of splitting your workouts, as it allows for minimum overlap between your workouts. The movements you do for push will not conflict with the movements you will do for pull. This ensures that all your muscles have a decent time to recover.

Let us look at more specific details of how you would structure these workouts. For each exercise that you do, you should do a small warm-up. Therefore, for each muscle, you would be doing two warm-ups and two exercises. When you are training your chest, for example, you might decide to do bench presses and pec decs (or chest flies). As a beginner, you should focus on reaching 10 reps (however, this can depend on what training you are doing, whether it be strength, endurance, or hypertrophy). You should do 10 reps for the warm-up, which is the same exercise but without weights—or extremely light ones. Then you would move onto 10 reps with a weight to bring you to failure at your desired rep; these are called 'working sets'. You would then do the same with pec dec, and then repeat for a certain amount of sets. In the same workout, you would be training your biceps. Therefore, you could do standing curls and hammer curls, and structure those exercises in the same way you did for your chest.

The difference between beginner and intermediate training is the frequency with which you train the same muscles. As the intensity of your workouts or the weights you are using increase, the frequency with which you train a body part each week should correspondingly decrease (Aceto, 2003). When you are a beginner, you are focusing more on the mind-to-muscle connection, practicing your form and your muscle coordination. You are also going to be using lighter weights. Because of this, your workout will be less intense—and less damaging to the body—so you will not need as long to recover your muscles before training them again. Furthermore, your body will respond to the smallest stimulus to your muscles simply because the movement is new. However, as your body gets used to what you are doing, you will need to increase the intensity and weights of your workouts to see progress. Because you are adding more weight, and therefore more stress to your muscles, you will need more time to recover. So, let's look at how you would move on to intermediate training.

If you are an intermediate, you should aim to train 4 days a week. You can start off on this split if you have been weightlifting for a while. You either do this by training for 4 days in a row and then taking two days off. So you would train Monday all the way through to Thursday and then take both Friday and Saturday off, then you repeat the cycle. This works well for bodybuilders, as this allows more time to pay attention to each body part.

The other option is to train for 2 days, take a rest day and then train for 2 days. So you would train on Monday and Tuesday, take a rest day on Wednesday, and then train again on Thursday and Friday. This also helps you with having more time to focus on each body part. Allowing for a rest day after every 2 days is also very beneficial because you have more time to train all your muscle groups, but this also allows you enough rest to go hard whenever you train. It gives you the energy to push yourself every day.

An example of this split would be to train chest and shoulders on Monday, legs and calves on Tuesday, arms and core on Thursday, and your back on Friday. Splitting your 4 days like this, no matter how you organize your rest days, is also good because it makes sure that you are not working arms 2 days in a row, which allows for better upper-body recovery.

Your main focus as you move on to intermediate training should be progressively increasing your weights and your intensity. Now that you have mastered the basics, you are going to see the most progress through progressive overload. This is when you gradually increase the weights or intensity in your routine in order to challenge your body and allow your musculoskeletal system to get stronger (Chertoff, 2020). This is the key to building strength and mass in your muscles. However, be sure to do this gradually. One of the biggest mistakes athletes make when trying to get stronger through progressive overload is making huge jumps, either in the weights they are using or in the number of reps they are doing. To see progress, you should focus on a gradual increase. Let's start with how to up your reps.

When you start your intermediate training split, your first working set should still be 10 reps. A working set means you are using weights to or near failure, so basically, a set that is not a warm-up. You should be using a weight that is heavy and challenging, yet you should be able to do 10 reps and be able to complete another 1–2 reps where you are strained, but do not need a spotter. You should then complete 1–2 more sets of 10 reps, but then time doing them in an accelerated and exploding fashion, as this helps to recruit an increased amount of muscle fibers (Aceto, 2003). After this, the key is to do reps until you reach failure, which could be anywhere between 6 and 10 reps.

These sets will require a spotter, and the key is that the last 2 reps should be extremely hard to finish. That is why a spotter is so important. When you switch to intermediate, it is important to focus on heavier weights and slightly fewer reps.

So, let's look at how you would work your chest for an intermediate split. Let's say for chest, you were using the bench press, as well as an incline bench press. For the bench press, you would do a warm-up with 10 reps, either with no weights or very light weights. You would then add weight and do 2-3 working sets for roughly 10 reps each. To finish off, you would do one set with increased weight, until you reach failure in approximately 6–10 reps. You would then repeat this with an incline bench press.

There is no clear and concise way to decide when to move from an intermediate training split to an advanced one. It could be after you find that you don't need as many recovery days, or that your body is not feeling as challenged by the intermediate split. This is a good indicator that maybe it is time to move onto the advanced split. It is important that your body is ready to train for 5 days a week. If you move on to this too quickly, you run the risk of overtraining, and you will see no progress. Overtraining is when you push your body too far and do not allow it time to recover. Rest is essential for muscle growth, both in size and strength. Overtraining undercuts that growth, so it is important to listen to your body. A good way to avoid overtraining is to progress slowly through how you split your workout. Listen to the signals your body is giving you to make sure it is ready to move on to an advanced split.

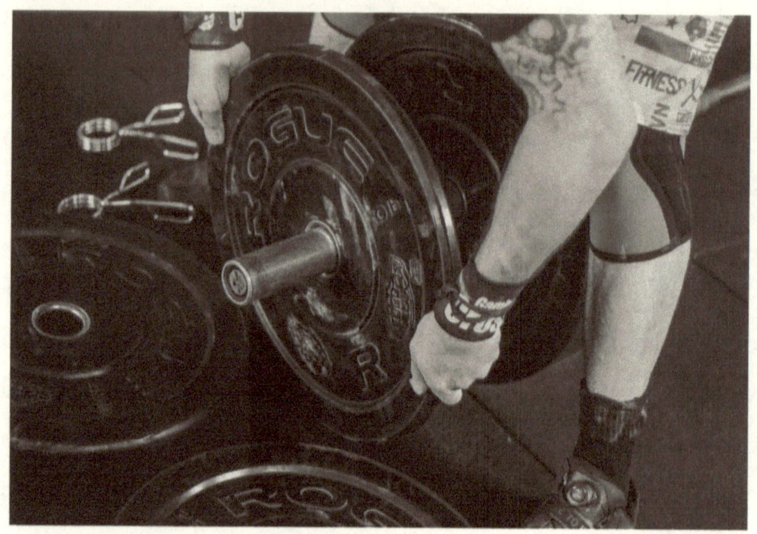

An advanced split allows for each body part to have a dedicated day, with 5 training days followed by 2 days of rest. This allows you to completely focus on one muscle at a time, and as we have said before, slow, deliberate, and focused training will always yield the best results. It also prevents you from spending long training sessions in the gym, which helps with growth. This might sound counterintuitive—surely the longer you spend in the gym, the more your muscles will grow. However, research has shown that long training sessions burn up large amounts of glycogen, the source of energy for your muscles. This process of using up the glycogen can inadvertently trigger the release of hormones that prevent your muscles from gaining size (Aceto, 2003). Therefore, only working on one muscle each training day is a good way to prevent this.

An example of an advanced split would be to train your back on Monday, your chest on Tuesday, your legs on Wednesday, your shoulders on Thursday, and your arms on Friday. You would then take a rest day for both Saturday and Sunday, and allow your muscles to recover. This is also good because it ensures that you are taking a full week's rest in between working the same muscle. There are other ways to break down the 5-day split. You can do the two on, one off method that was mentioned during the intermediate split, and still focus on one muscle group per day. You might find that interspersing your rest days like that yields better results for you.

There are a number of tips that can help you move from intermediate to advanced training and deal with the progressive increase in weights throughout your journey. The key is to do reps until you reach failure, and you should be reaching between at least 6 and 10 reps for each set. However, to guide yourself into this while still pushing your muscles, you can do things like rest-pauses and stripped sets.

A rest-pause is when you take a short break, no longer than 20 seconds, in between reps. Let's say you are using the bench press and aiming for 8 reps. Maybe you only manage to get 6. You would then rest the weight for 10–20 seconds before finishing off the last 2 reps.

Another way to push yourself is to do strip sets also know as drop sets, which allows you to start with a very heavy weight and slowly lower it as you reach failure. You start with a heavy set of dumbbells and aim for 10 reps. When you reach failure at 5 reps, swap the dumbbells for a slightly lighter pair. When you can only achieve maybe 3 reps with these, switch to an even lighter pair and do the last 2 reps, at which point you should reach failure with those (Aceto, 2003). Light strip sets do not cause maximal failure; therefore you need to push yourself and start with weights with which you can barely manage 4–5 reps. It is through this repetitive failure that you will see progress. Just because you cannot complete something perfectly does not mean it is not working. You should be struggling, as that is a sign that you are working your muscles to their full capacity. All of these techniques ensure that you reach your limit—and manage to push even further!

As previously mentioned, the key to progress is progressive overload and heavy weights. One of the biggest mistakes that many people make is using weights that are too light. If your weights are too light, you are not recruiting all of your muscle fibers, and you are therefore unlikely to make significant progress.

Effective progressive overload means a gradual increase in weights. The smallest increase in weight can make the biggest difference. Do not go from leg pressing 180 lbs one week to 225 lbs the next. Your reps are unlikely to be clean, with your form and muscle coordination suffering. Your legs might also become too sore and you may not be able to continue your training without a long recovery period. Sticking to smaller jumps is smarter and more productive, as it does not shock the muscle. It allows for complete recovery, as well as time for your muscles to adapt. Therefore, it is smarter to go up in small increments every week, even if you feel you could do more. So instead of jumping from 180 to 225 lbs, try to go up to 190 or 195 lbs. And then the week after that, go up by another 5 or 10 lbs, and so on.

Furthermore, if you jump straight up to 225 lbs and find it too heavy, the next workout you might scale back to 210 lbs. This is not progressive overload. The whole point is to achieve a gradual increase, not to continually go up and down in your weights. If you increase in smaller amounts, you can be sure that you can handle the increase in weight and you will not have to go back and forth. Slow and steady wins the race in this case.

The most important thing to remember as you go on this fitness journey is to have patience. This is not a sprint that you are embarking on, it is a marathon. It is something that you should start with the intention of sustaining throughout your life. You may not start to see the kind of progress you want after a week or two, but if you stick with it, you will see the beginning of that progress within a matter of months. It is important to move through this plan slowly, from beginner to advanced, as your muscles allow it. You will see the most progress this way. The most important things to remember when planning your workouts are to focus on slowly increasing weight and intensity, to focus on correct form and coordination, and to find a balance between pushing your body beyond its limits and damaging it. This chapter shows you how to find that balance.

CHAPTER 6: MAXIMIZE YOUR WORKOUTS

———— ◆ ◇ ◆ ————

When you first start lifting, everything is going to be challenging for you. You are using your muscles in ways they have never been used before, and because you are continually challenging them, your progress is going to be rapid. You will feel your muscle soreness after your workouts and you will see the increase in both your muscle strength and mass in very clear ways. Progress is also easier and more obvious because you are moving from nothing.

However, as you continue on this journey, you might find yourself hitting a plateau where you see and feel very little progress. A plateau is when your body "adjusts to the demands of your workout" (Sweat, 2019). You will find yourself at a point in your journey where you feel like you have hit a wall. The human body is built for adaptation, and therefore it will eventually train itself to easily tackle whatever you throw at it during your workouts.

In order to see progress, you have to struggle. It is the same reason you increase training days and your weights progressively: Once your muscles are used to a certain intensity and weight, it no longer challenges them, therefore they do not grow or become stronger. It may seem inevitable that you will always eventually hit plateaus, however, there are several ways to avoid them and continually maximize your workouts. This is how you will continually see the best results.

One of the best ways to get the most out of your workouts and avoid plateaus is to continually shock your system. Plateaus happen because your muscles get used to the movement and the weight. However, if you are changing up the way you challenge them, this is not going to happen. While the most common way we do this is to increase the weight, after a while, your body will become accustomed to this too. So, we have to get a bit more creative with it, and there are so many ways to do this that not enough weightlifters know about or use.

You can change the speed of your reps. You can make them slower, or do paused reps instead of regular ones. Or you can make the movements more difficult by changing the angle with which you perform your lifts. You can also change up how you do your sets, both through doing drop sets and supersets, and essentially changing either how long you rest in between sets and the intensity of the set itself. Another way to maximize your workouts is by changing how you fuel yourself for them, by focusing on your carb intake and your level of hydration.

One of the first ways you can maximize your workouts is to change up the speed of your reps. You can increase the intensity of a rep simply by slowing it down. Going too quickly through your reps is far less effective in building muscle and seeing progress than moving slowly through them. Think about it. If you blow through 12 reps quickly in a matter of seconds and then spend 10 minutes resting and checking your social media, do you think your muscles have been put under strain? It is far more effective if you slow the reps down. Each time you lift, make sure you are taking a few seconds to pull it up. Hold it at the top for a moment and then take your time to lower it down. Make sure each rep is about 10 seconds in total. This increases the time your muscle is under tension and makes a huge difference in whether you feel the exercise or not. On the other side of the coin if you have always worked with slow reps speed them up a little.

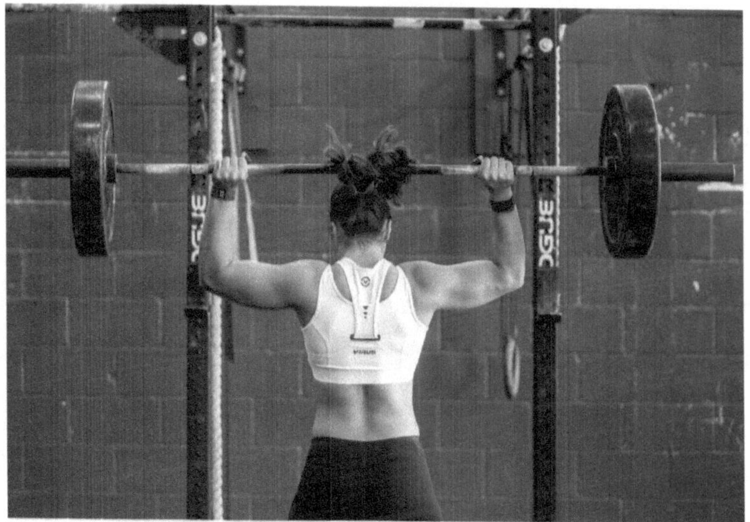

Another way to slow down your movement is to do pause reps. Pause reps are exactly what they sound like—at some point during your rep, you stop and hold the weight for as long as you want. You can do this during the concentric or eccentric part of the movement, and hold it for anywhere from 3 to 30 seconds, depending on how many reps you are doing and how well you can handle the weight. For example, when you are bench pressing, you can push the weight up and hold it at the top. Or you can pause when the weight is lowered just above your chest. Start off with weights that are roughly 70–80% of your one-rep max and do around 3 sets of 5 reps each. When you first attempt this, start on the lighter side and then slowly build your way up. This will help you to avoid injury and know where your limits are. Pause reps work your muscles harder for the same reason slowed down reps do—you cannot rely on momentum to complete the rep. It is engaging all your muscles to hold that weight there. It increases the force you have to exert, as well as the extent and time your muscles are under tension. This greatly increases your strength without having to increase your weight and helps you to further perfect your form.

Beyond speed, there are other ways that you can increase the difficulty of your reps in order to feel them more. The key to changing up your routine is to find new ways to push yourself and challenge your muscles. One way to do this is forced reps. This is a variation that will require a partner, as someone needs to spot you. Forced reps are when you continue to do reps past your point of failure. The forced reps are the ones you do when you are out of steam, and a partner can help you to complete them by picking up the slack (Heyer, 2019). So, let's say that you aim for 8 reps, but you chose a weight that you can only lift cleanly for 6 clean reps. You then have a spotter to help you to get the last 2 reps, and this places even more stress on muscles that have already failed. You can also do forced reps by yourself, but only if your gym as foot assisted machines or you are doing say single arm machine curls use your free hand to assist. Do not attempt to do these using barbells. You can do this by maximizing your time under tension and taking your time to slowly lower the weights when going through the eccentric movement.

Not all exercises can be comfortably and safely done with forced reps. You shouldn't attempt this with exercises like deadlifts, dips, lunges, or barbell rows. It would be awkward and almost impossible for a spotter to help complete reps on those exercises after you have failed. However, forced reps work well for many of the classic exercises. You can do them when you are doing bench presses, bicep curls, shoulder presses, and tricep extensions. The main thing to remember is caution, and make sure that your spotter (if you have one) is on board with what you want to do.

Forced reps work to build muscle mass and strength because they continue to place the already failed muscle under strain, and ensure that 100% of the muscles you are targeting are working.

They fatigue more muscle fiber than those already in use. Furthermore, it allows you to get more volume into your set at a more challenging weight. Instead of only being able to do 5 reps, you can now do 8 for every set.

It is important that just the right amount of resistance is being transferred from you to your spotter. They should assist just enough that you can continue at the same rate as before; you should still be doing most of the work. Once the spotter is doing more of the work, you should stop. This is why using a spotter you trust is so important. Too much help and you won't be doing the right amount of work, too little and you will not be able to go through with the reps. Forced reps are an excellent way to mix up your workout and add a different form of intensity to your muscles that can help to lift you out of a plateau.

Another way to push your muscles and change up your routine is to do drop sets. Drop sets are about working out until failure and not allowing rest. The idea is that you do one set with a heavy weight until failure, at which point you drop those weights, pick up slightly lighter weights and do another set. You can do this for several sets, going down in weight each time. You can do this with any exercise or drills, and there are even several ways you can do it. You can choose one weight and then lift until failure, then drop to a lower weight and do another set until failure, and then drop again. You can do as many sets of this as you like. Or you can plan to complete a specific number of reps before dropping down to a lower weight. For example, you could plan to do bicep curls for 10 reps with 40 lbs, then 10 reps with 30 lbs, and then another 10 reps with 20 lbs (Baur, 2011).

Drop sets work because dropping to lighter weights helps to recruit muscle fibers that otherwise wouldn't be activated if you stayed at the same weight. An important part of feeling drop sets is to not rest in between sets. If you rest for more than 10 seconds, you will not feel the full burn of these variations in your muscles. Another way to do this is to change the amount of weight that you drop between sets. The general standard is to drop by 20% each time, but you can change this depending on what you feel challenges you. It is also a good idea to have the weights you plan to use at the ready, because then you spend less time getting ready between each set and can keep up the pace that this type of training demands. By pushing your muscles beyond the point of failure each time with a lighter weight, you are recruiting all your muscle fibers and you will therefore see considerable growth in both strength and mass.

It is important to exercise caution with all of these variations, but particularly with drop sets. Because you are doing more reps and not resting in between sets, you run the risk of causing injury or overtraining. You are essentially trying to shock your muscles into a new period of growth, and therefore it would be unwise to overdo it. First, you should start with lower weights than you would usually use. This is mostly because you will be doing more reps, which will test your endurance. For example, if you usually bench press 180 lbs for 10 reps, drop that down to at least 140 lbs. You can go down even further—start low and bump up the weight to find your limit rather than start above your limit and risk an injury. It is also wise to limit the number of drop sets you include in your routine. Do not use it for every exercise and every set, rather use it for one exercise per muscle group. So, if you are working your chest, do drop sets for the bench press but then do normal sets for pec decs or your incline bench press. If you use this variation too much, you will overtrain and you will not see any results. However, if you are smart about the way you implement this technique into your routine, you will not have to worry about falling into plateaus again.

Another way to maximize your workouts and challenge your muscles is to simply change the angle at which you lift. If you change the angle of many of your basic exercises, you will find that the shift puts stress on slightly different muscle fibers than you are used to. Using different angles can cause different "patterns of contraction" within the same muscles (Aceto, 2003). For example, you can change where you place your feet when you do leg presses. You will feel a difference in the way the machine works your leg depending on how far apart your feet are, or how high they are on the machine. Another example is heel-raised squats. Place two weight plates under your heels when doing your squats and watch how you start to feel different muscles in your quads and glutes that you didn't know that you had! Pointing your toes inward or outward for deadlifts will also work slightly different muscles in your hamstrings and glutes. Changing the angles and positions that you use when you work out is a simple but effective way to add variety into your current workout routine and push yourself out of a plateau. The best part is that you can play around with angels and see what works for you.

The final variation we will look at is supersets. Supersets are essentially switching between different exercises without allowing any rest in between. Supersets have a number of benefits. They push your muscles and allow you to work different muscle groups at the same time while still achieving fatigue in both. It is good for maintaining balance in your body and improves your muscular endurance or tenacity. It also provides a significant challenge for your muscles because of the change in routine and because rest time between sets is limited. It is a great variation to add to your weekly routine in order to force your muscles out of a possible plateau. Furthermore, you do not run as great a risk of overtraining as you do with other workout variations. You can therefore do supersets with all your muscle groups throughout the week, or just use it once or twice during your workouts to provide some variation. Either way you do it, you will see progress. They also tend to take less time than traditional sets, therefore, you might find them very helpful if you're short on time on certain days of the week. You are still getting the same workout; it just requires a lot less of your time.

There are different types of supersets, depending on how you want to group your exercises. The most common kind is agonist or antagonistic sets. This is when you combine two exercises that use two different muscle groups (Boly, 2017). The idea is to avoid fatigue and overtraining a specific muscle group. So, if you were doing your back and chest on the same day, you could alternate between one chest exercise and one back exercise for each superset. For example, the first superset could be bench press and dumbbell rows. This is beneficial because it allows you to go heavy with each exercise, straining each muscle group, while also wearing yourself out. It also allows you to create a balanced body in a limited time.

The next type of superset involves working the same muscle group and is known as post-activation potentiation (PAP) training. This is when you train the same muscle group or do similar movements, and is most beneficial when aiming to induce muscular hypertrophy. Because of that, it is ideal for muscle growth. An example of this would be to do a bench press and then a light tricep push down. If you wanted to make your workout more complex, you could add dynamic movement. For example, you could do a set of weighted squats, and then a set of explosive box jumps. Doing this causes much more strain on your muscles, which can stimulate muscle growth.

The last kind of supersets combines an upper body and a lower body movement. This can be beneficial if you are training your full body in one workout, but it is not one that I would recommend if you want to see significant progress. An example of this would be to superset walking lunges with pull-ups. It can be helpful for muscular endurance, but overall, the first two styles of supersets are far more suited to the average athlete's goals.

When it comes to supersets, it is often wise to do shorter sets with heavy weights. If you are only achieving failure after 12 reps or more for each exercise, you are focusing more on muscle endurance than strength and growth. If you want to increase muscle mass, it is often better to do no more than 12 reps total in each set. So, if you were doing legs, for example, you would do 6 reps on the leg press and then 6 reps of squats. With supersets, you should not feel the need to lower the weights as you will be doing approximately the same number of reps. It is challenging more because of the lack of rest in between exercises.

Lastly, let's look at how you are fueling yourself for your workouts. If our bodies are not properly prepared for our workouts, we may not be able to push ourselves to our peak. It's like driving a car on an empty tank; it makes no sense! We are not going to see progress and we are going to plateau. If you have not mastered fueling your body with carbohydrates and water before a workout, trying out any of the other tips in this chapter is almost pointless.

Carbohydrates often have a bad reputation, but they are essential for an energized and effective workout. Ideally, you should get in some kind of carb roughly half an hour before your workout. It also helps to combine your carbs with a lean protein. This does not mean you have to eat a full meal, as this is likely to make you sluggish. Instead, opt for a snack. A banana is always a good choice, and you can have it with some kind of nut butter in order to add protein. You could opt for any fruit or vegetables, low-fat yogurt, or whole grain options, such as whole wheat toast or cereals. All of these would be good options. When you eat carbohydrates, they break down into smaller sugars, such as glucose and fructose, and those not used for immediate tasks are converted into glycogen and stored in the muscles. When you work out immediately after eating these foods, your muscles are full of glycogen, which is ready to be used for exercise (Quinn, 2007). Because it has just been stored, it is immediately accessible. Eating carbohydrates is essential for maximizing your workouts, for feeling your most energized during your session, and therefore, for making decent progress.

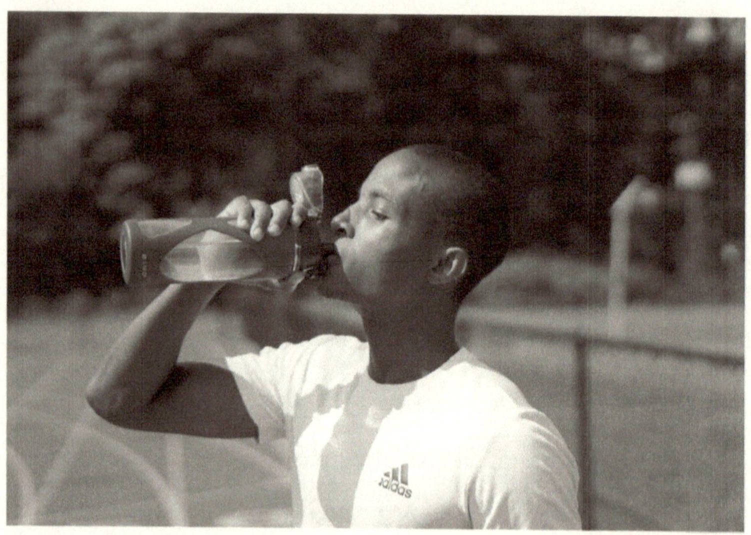

Hydration is often underestimated in its ability to dictate the success of your workouts. Simply put, if you are not hydrating enough before, during, and after your workouts, you are depriving your muscles of water and risking dehydration. Water is important because it regulates your body temperature and lubricates your joints, both of which help to prevent injury. It also helps to carry nutrients and energy throughout the body. If you are not hydrated, you will not feel energized during your workout. You also might experience symptoms such as dizziness, cramps, and fatigue.

If you are not hydrated, your body cannot perform at its highest level and you will be unable to get the most out of your workouts. It is important to drink at least 2 liters (or about 8–10 glasses) of water each day. If you are exercising, your body is also sweating and getting rid of the water, so it is even more important to hydrate. You should drink at least 20 ounces over the 2–3 hours before you start exercising, with 8 ounces of that volume consumed 20–30 minutes before your workout. During your workout, you should drink 8 ounces every 10–20 minutes. Then, you should drink another 8 ounces in the 30 minutes after you finish working out (American Academy of Family Physicians, 2010). If you do not drink enough water, your progress will be halted because you cannot push yourself enough to see changes.

It is natural to reach plateaus in our fitness journey. Our muscles are excellent at adapting, so if you are not constantly changing up your routine, they are going to adapt to how you exercise them and they will stop progressing. You need to add variety in order to see consistent progress—you need to find new ways to move, that shock your system and push it. By using the techniques outlined in this chapter, you will be able to avoid plateaus throughout your fitness journey and will never stop seeing progress. Some of these tips, such as fueling yourself with carbs and water, will be something that you will use every week in your fitness routine. However, some techniques you may use for a brief period and then switch to something else. Once you find yourself getting used to your routine, you should change it up. Maybe try drop sets for a month in some of your exercises, and then spend a month trying out supersets. Maybe rotate the variations out by the week. Maybe supersets are something that will become a regular feature in your routine, and you occasionally use pause reps and drop sets. The way you chose to do it isn't important—what is important is that your routine is constantly changing. That is how you maximize your workouts.

CHAPTER 7: EVERYTHING SUPPLEMENTS

When you think of how you fuel your body, the first thing that you are likely to think of is your food. And you would be right! Food is where you are going to get the majority of what you need in terms of nutrition, vitamins, and macros. However, in order to maximize your workouts, you need to maximize how you supply your body. While supplements such as vitamins and protein powders are not essential, they will enable you to push yourself. They are what is going to set you apart from the average athlete. They will help you to build your ideal physique by reducing your body fat and maximizing your muscle gain. They will help you to stay motivated and energized and build your strength.

With so many options for supplements, it can be hard to know where to start. They will all benefit you in different ways, so deciding what you want to use is just a matter of sorting out what your goals are, and taking what is needed to help you achieve them. As overwhelming as it can seem, I am going to make it incredibly simple. In this chapter, I am going to outline all the supplements, what you would take them for, and how they benefit your workouts. You will simply decide from there which ones are right for you. So, let's get started with everything supplements!

Protein Powder

Undoubtedly, one of the first supplements that comes to mind when we talk about fitness is protein powder. It comes in a couple of different forms, and you have probably seen protein powder, protein bars, and protein drinks in stores and advertised on TV. Protein is one of the most popular dietary supplements, as it helps muscles to recover and repair themselves, which lends itself to muscle growth in both strength and mass. However, there is an overwhelming number of options when it comes to protein supplements. So let's unpack them.

When it comes to protein powder, there are a couple of different variations that you can get. First, let's focus on the three different types of basic protein powders: whey, egg, and plant-based. When it comes to choosing between these three, the most common factor will be your existing diet and preferences.

The first and most popular one is, of course, whey protein. Whey protein is so popular because it is affordable, accessible, and effective. Whey protein is a by-product from the cheese and yogurt making process. In order to make cheese or yogurt, milk is curdled. The curds are then strained and made into either cheese or yogurt, and the liquid that is left behind from the straining contains fat-digesting proteins that are commonly known as whey (Tinsley, 2017). This is made into a powder, which is how we get whey protein powder. It is considered highly effective because once you consume it, whey is rapidly and easily digested by the body. Therefore, it gets into your bloodstream and your muscles very quickly, so the recovery and repair of your muscles happens efficiently. Whey also contains all the amino acids that your body requires. Over all the other proteins, whey is considered the most effective because it also helps to produce new protein in your muscles. This helps the repair and recovery process move along even more quickly, which aids in muscle growth in mass and strength.

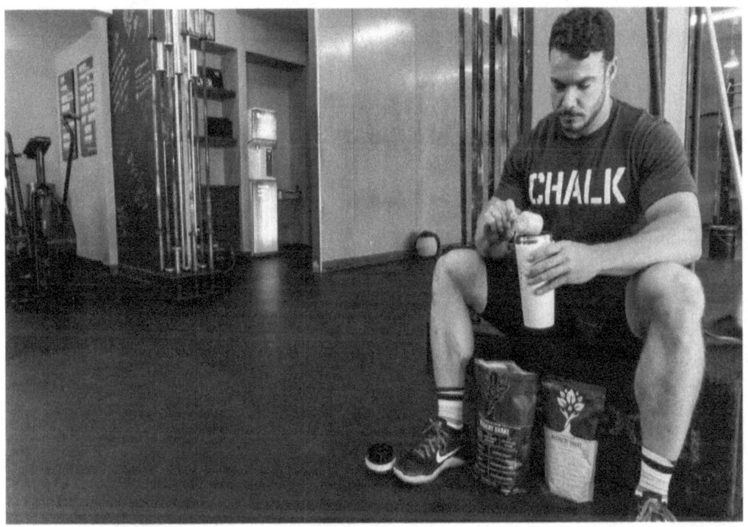

There are also two different kinds of whey proteins: whey isolates and whey concentrates. They differ both in how they are made and how they benefit you. The main difference in their production is how much processing they go through. When the liquid whey is collected after the cheese-making process, it still undergoes several types of processing to increase its level of protein. After a sufficient level of protein is reached, the liquid can be dried to form whey concentrate. The macros of whey concentrate work out to approximately 80% protein by weight. The remaining 20% consists of carbohydrates and fats.

On the other hand, isolate whey undergoes several more levels of processing and ends up with 90% of its weight as protein (Tinsley, 2017). Therefore, isolate whey is slightly higher in protein, while lower in carbs and lactose. However, whey isolate is more expensive and the amino acids found in both are almost identical.

Whether you choose whey concentrate or whey isolate is dependent on your goals and how much money you would like to spend. If you are not too fussy about the level of carbs and are looking to spend less, it would make more sense to go for whey concentrate. However, if you are trying to lose fat and cut carbs, the whey isolate may be more suited to your goals. Also, if you are lactose intolerant, it might be wiser to go for the whey isolate. However, both forms tend to be safe enough for lactose-intolerant people to consume, unless you are particularly sensitive.

Another type of protein to take into account is caseins protein. Casein is the other type of protein that comes from dairy byproducts and is a slow-release protein. Casein is the main type of protein found in dairy products and makes up about 80% of the protein found in cow's milk. You can buy casein protein powder supplements, but you can also get it from whole foods, such as greek yogurt or cottage cheese (Harris-Fry, 2018). Whey digests and gets into your muscles almost immediately, however casein protein releases the amino acids slowly. This is because casein is more gel-forming in the gut, so it slows down the digestion process.

Another form of protein is egg protein, which is a powder made from separated and dehydrated egg whites. It is beneficial because it is a complete protein source, which means it has all the necessary amino acids, as well as several vitamins and minerals that will benefit your health. However, it is more expensive and not as tasty, with limited flavors and options.

There are also a number of plant-based proteins to choose from if you are vegan, vegetarian, or even particularly sensitive to lactose. Some people find that whey powder makes them break out or upsets their stomach, so plant-based options are a great option for them.

There are several plant-based protein powders to consider as alternatives. One of the most popular is pea protein, made from golden peas. It is a slow-release protein like caseins, and is therefore best to take at night, as it releases amino acids gradually. It is a good vegan alternative, however, it is not a complete protein source, so you can't rely on it alone. A better option for a complete plant-based protein might be soy protein. Soy is hulled, dried in a powder, and then concentrated or isolated in a protein powder. It is one of the few plant-based proteins that contains all the amino acids and is relatively reasonable in price. However, if you are a woman, it can cause you to gain weight. It contains high levels of estrogen, which can cause increased fat storage (Warner, 2014). Furthermore, some people can be allergic to soy. If you are a vegan or have soy, dairy, or gluten allergies, the best option would be rice protein. Brown rice contains high levels of proteins, which are then isolated and ground into a powder. It is a decent alternative and does contain B vitamins, however, it is not a complete protein source and does not have all the necessary amino acids.

No matter what your goal, protein is an essential part of your diet. Whether you are aiming to lose fat, gain mass or muscle, or anything in between, you will see the best results in your workouts and your body by including protein in your diet. If you are doing any kind of physical activity, it is important to increase your protein intake, and protein powders are a quick and effective way to do that if obtaining the protein from food alone is not possible. However, different kinds of proteins are good for different times of the day. Post-workout, the ideal protein to ingest is whey protein. Whey protein digests quickly and immediately finds its way into your muscle, which is important for recovery immediately after a workout. It is recommended that you have whey protein within 30 minutes of your workout ending. On the other hand, you should take casein protein powder just before you go to bed. Because it is slow-release, it essentially drips-feeds amino acids into your bloodstream and muscles as you sleep. This helps to rebuild muscle tissue overnight. Pea protein is also slow-release so you could also take it just before you go to bed.

Carb Powders

The next kind of supplement that you might consider including in your diet is carb powder. As we've said before, carbohydrates are energy. They are equal in importance to protein in making sure that your workouts are their most effective. While protein is something you need after a workout to help your muscles recover, carbs are something you need to take before, and sometimes during, a workout to ensure that your muscles have enough energy in the first place. Carbs have a number of benefits, such as increased performance during workouts, as well as an increase in growth of muscle mass.

Carbs are beneficial for energy, as they can be converted to adenosine triphosphate (ATP), which is the only form of energy that causes your muscles to contract and forces them to lift. However, your body uses up the ATP stored in its muscle within a few seconds of lifting. When your ATP has run out, your body switches to using the process of glycolysis, which is when your body uses glycogen and blood sugar to replace the store of ATP in the muscles. The only way to supply your muscles with enough glycogen to do this is to eat carbs. If you eat some form of carbohydrates before or during your workout, it converts to glycogen that is stored in your muscles or immediately goes through glycolysis to convert the blood sugar into ATP (Campbell et al., 2008). If you do not have a sufficient amount of carbs in your body, you will not physically have the energy to continuously lift heavy weights during your workouts. If you cannot train hard for the duration of your workouts, you will not see progress or growth. Carbohydrates are essential for that.

Beyond our performance in the gym, carbohydrates are good in the long run for muscle growth and retention. This is mainly due to insulin. Consuming carbs causes your body to release insulin, which is key in both building muscle mass and retaining it. Insulin supports muscle growth because it increases the transport of amino acids around the body. It is also anti-catabolic, which means it helps to prevent muscle loss, as it reduces the effects of cortisol in the blood. Cortisol breaks down muscle and converts it to energy. However, if insulin levels are high, cortisol levels are low, so it prevents muscle loss.

While it is important to get the majority of your carbohydrates from foods, just like with protein, supplements can boost the levels of carbohydrates in your diet in a quick and effective way. One of the best uses for carb supplements is to get carbs during your workout, also known as intra-workout carbs. This helps to prevent fatigue during exercise. It provides immediate fuel, replacing the glycogen stores in the muscles that can then be converted to ATP to help you continue lifting (Salter, 2016). Consuming carb supplements throughout your workouts ensures that you can give your all for however long you're lifting. You won't experience dips, as your muscles will be continually fueled. It is essential for pushing your body and getting results.

Pre-Workout

One of the biggest problems people often have is finding the energy to work out. I'm sure you have felt that way before—maybe it's the end of a long workday, or maybe you just can't manage to crawl your way out of bed at 5 a.m. some mornings. You know you need to go to the gym, but you're so low on energy and working out is the last thing in the world that you feel like doing. What if I told you that you don't need to summon the will power and the giant push of energy to drive to the gym and start the workout all by yourself? You just need enough energy to take some pre-workout and you'll get the little boost you need to take you the rest of the way.

Pre-workout is a supplement that you take before you work out that gives you energy. There are several benefits to taking pre-workout before you lift. It improves your energy levels, motivation, stamina, and focus. It also helps you to maintain energy, and studies have shown that caffeine causes 66% more glycogen to stay in your muscles after your workout, which promotes muscle growth. Some kinds of pre-workout contain caffeine, and caffeine, itself, also has a number of benefits. Caffeine has been shown to block off the pain as you work out, which allows you to focus on pushing harder (M Club, 2017).

There are two different types of pre-workouts to look out for: stimulant-based pre-workouts and non-stimulant-based pre-workouts. Stim-based pre-workouts contain ingredients that stimulate the nervous system. On the other hand, non-stim pre-workouts do not contain stimulants that affect your nervous system. They provide a pump to your muscles, energy, and endurance, without any of the neurological effects (String, 2014).

The biggest difference between these two types is the inclusion of caffeine. Most non-stim pre-workouts do not contain caffeine, while most stim-pre-workouts contain large amounts.

Some contain so much that it can be a very bad idea to take more than the recommended serving size. While this may sound scary, it is often not harmful if you follow the recommendations. You are going to find way more benefits from taking pre-workout with stimulants than without. However, you also might benefit from alternating between the two types.

Stim-based pre-workouts are the cause behind many of the problems that some people experience with pre-workout. There are a variety of cons that you might encounter, most notably insomnia, if you take it too late at night. This is, of course, due to the high levels of caffeine. If you take stim-based pre-workout too often, it can be overstimulating and you can become addicted to it and you might find that you cannot workout without it. It can also cause adrenal fatigue and dehydration if you are not drinking enough water. Beta-alanine, which is found in stim-based pre-workout and non-stim pre-workout, can also cause your face to itch. This is not harmful, but can be quite disconcerting if you are not expecting it. These problems can be avoided by taking pre-workout in moderation. Don't take it every day, just a few times a week. Try to take it when you really need a push in energy, maybe after a long week or a hard day at work. It should be a tool that helps you to work out to your best, not something that you are dependent upon.

Vitamins and Fish Oil

There are a few supplements you can add into your daily routine that will benefit your overall health, which in turn will help your training. First and foremost is the multivitamin, a supplement that contains high concentrations of at least 13 vitamins and 25 minerals that are essential to your health (Carter, 2019). The nutrients contained in multivitamins are beneficial for the general maintenance and functioning of your body. They help with cardiovascular health, strengthening the immune system, reproductive health in women, and the regulation of the body and cellular function. This is important when it comes to maintaining an optimal workout routine; your body has to be functioning at its peak. It will also help with muscle growth and maintenance. While you will get most of these vitamins from a balanced diet, taking a multivitamin can often help to boost these levels and ensure they are optimal.

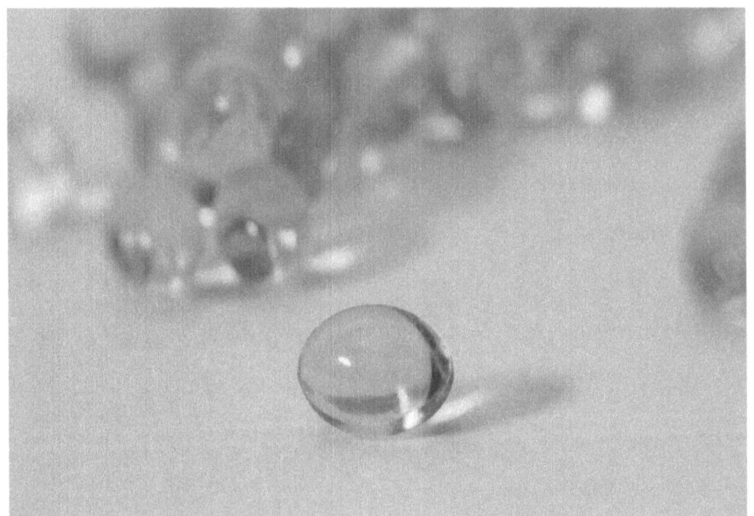

Another optional supplement that is beneficial for you is fish oil, which is high in omega-3 fatty acids. You can find omega-3 fatty acids in high levels in fish, such as mackerel, tuna, and anchovies. However, if you do not get 1-2 servings of fish per week, fish oil supplements are a good way to bridge that gap in your diet. It is an important part of your diet because it lubricates and aids in the preservation of joints (Robertson, 2018). This is especially beneficial when it comes to weightlifting, as heavy weights commonly cause injuries in the lifter's joints before anything else. Omega-3 supplements can help to prevent that and ensure that you can continue to work hard without worrying about damaging your joints and halting your training routine. It can aid with weight or fat loss and can improve bone health.

While supplements are a huge aid to working out, they can never replace the real thing. Carb and protein supplements are invaluable for maximizing your energy and muscle growth and repair, however, eating foods high in those macronutrients is far more important. Supplements are quick and easy ways to get these nutrients into your body, but the best thing you can do for yourself is to create a base of a balanced diet. Your diet takes up your entire day—every decision that you make about food from the time you wake up to the time you go to sleep can either contribute to your fitness goals or hinder them. You cannot make poor food choices throughout the day and fix them with supplements. You need to be eating whole foods, balanced meals, and smart snacks consistently, with a healthy balance of carbohydrates, fats, protein, and vitamins. Supplements are merely a way to give you that extra boost.

CHAPTER 8: THE ENDLESS BENEFITS OF REST AND RECOVERY

We've looked at how to push your body to its limits, but you only do that for a few hours a day, at most. So what makes up the rest of your time? Recovery and care. Once you have annihilated your muscles at the gym in the morning, you have to spend the rest of the day making sure that they have the adequate tools to repair and subsequently grow.

The necessity of rest and recovery is often overlooked by many people during the span of their fitness journey. It is assumed that the best way to see results is to push yourself and your muscles to the brink of exhaustion every day, perhaps for hours. However, our bodies will not become strong that way. If our bodies are a machine, continually running them to their max every day is going to cause them to deteriorate and break down at a rapid rate. We would be unwise to overuse the machine without allowing time for it to be repaired. We need to do the same with our bodies and our training. Rest days are an essential part of maximizing your workouts.

One of the biggest threats to progress is overtraining. The first sign of overtraining is overreaching. This is when the typical post-workout muscle soreness is persistent, and you do not allow enough time to rest and recover that soreness between your workouts. If you ignore overreaching and keep going, you will hit overtraining. This is harder to reverse and may take weeks or months to come back from. You are essentially breaking down your body to the point of no return. You will know you have overtrained when you start to feel weaker consistently, and your performance is constantly lacking, as you cannot lift as heavy weights as you could before. Your progress will plateau, and it will take far longer for your muscles to recover. You will also feel overwhelming fatigue in your everyday life, and you will struggle to sleep and feel moody (Women's Sport Medical Centre, 2018).

When you have reached this point, you need to stop and rest, sometimes for weeks. You need to reevaluate your diet and your routine, and when you do return, you have to do it slowly. By not taking rest into account, you are risking taking weeks off training and pushing back your progress all the way to the beginning. The key to avoiding overtraining is good sleep, rest days, and looking into things such as deep tissue or active release therapy.

Sleep

Sleep is one of the most important tools we have at our disposal for maximizing our workouts. Sleep is the cornerstone to a healthy life. It would not matter if you followed every other trick and tip in this book to a tee—if you do not focus on getting the optimal amount of sleep, you will never reach your full fitness potential. You need to be consistent in your sleep and get enough hours. It needs to be uninterrupted and good quality sleep. This will help you with muscle growth and recovery. There are even benefits to taking small naps throughout the day.

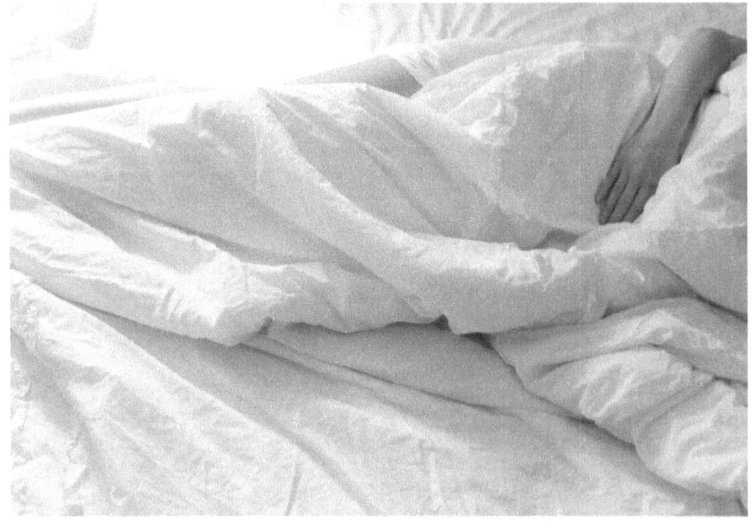

The good news is that you are more likely to sleep better when you are training consistently. Doing moderate to vigorous exercise a few times a week has been shown to improve sleep quality by decreasing the amount of time needed to fall asleep, also known as sleep onset, as well as decreasing the number of times you wake up and the length of time you stay awake during the night. Studies have shown that people who exercise at least three times a week are less likely to suffer from sleeping disorders, such as insomnia, sleep apnea, or restless leg syndrome. People who get regular exercise are also more likely to sleep more than six hours and experience better sleep quality

(Wunsch et al., 2017). While sleep may come easier to you because you are exercising, you still have to consciously make sure you are getting good sleep. The benefits are endless, and you will see your training progress skyrocket as a result.

Sleep is essential for your overall health—it improves your memory and cognitive abilities, as well as your mood. It also helps to regulate your blood sugar, your blood pressure, and prevents a number of different issues, including heart disease. Sleep is also important for weight maintenance and loss, as a decent amount of sleep enables you to make healthy food choices. If you are trying to eat healthy in order to support your training, or you are aiming to lose weight, not getting enough sleep will sabotage your attempts. Being sleep-deprived messes with the hormones in your brain that help to regulate your appetite, called leptin and ghrelin. When you are sleep-deprived, your appetite is less regulated, so you are going to eat more than you need. You also will tend to reach for less healthy options for comfort (Rachel Reiff Ellis, 2019). Combine this with working out less frequently or for shorter periods because you are tired, and you are very likely to gain weight and fat if you are not sleeping well.

Sufficient sleep is essential for your workouts as it gives you the energy you need to do them. It is near impossible to train hard when you are struggling to stay awake throughout the day. However, it is also important for the aftermath. Recovery and growth are boosted by sleep, and excessive sleep deprivation often hinders muscle growth. When you do not get enough sleep, you don't get the maximum replenishment of glycogen in the muscles. Sleep is one of the key times when the body converts the glucose in your blood to glycogen, which, as we know, the muscles use for fuel. If you are not sleeping enough, your muscles have less glycogen, so that they cannot grow and develop as quickly.

Furthermore, your muscles need sleep in order to release human growth hormone (HGH), as well as to undergo protein synthesis (International Sport Science Association, 2019). HGH is a hormone that is released during the non-REM part of your sleep cycle. REM (rapid-eye movement) sleep happens in cycles of about 90–120 minutes throughout the night and is responsible for restoring your mind. Non-REM sleep is known as 'deep sleep' and is the phase responsible for repair and recovery for the body and your muscles. It is during this phase that HGH is secreted. This growth hormone stimulates muscle repair and tissue growth. It is also responsible for breaking down the amino acids in the protein that we consume and using that to build up our muscles. If you do not sleep enough, your body does not secrete enough of the human growth hormone, and you are at risk of losing muscle mass instead of gaining it. In fact, it has been proven that no matter your food intake or exercise regime, sleep deprivation is likely to cause muscle shrinkage (International Sport Science Association, 2019).

The recommended amount of sleep for the average person is between 7 and 9 hours per night. You might find that you function better on 7 hours than on 9 hours. However, athletes tend to need more sleep for recovery. Therefore, you might need closer to 9 or 10 hours to feel properly rested. Sticking to a consistent sleep schedule is also key. You should be falling asleep and waking up at roughly the same times every day. It also needs to be uninterrupted sleep. If you are waking up frequently, you will not feel well rested.

Your level of activity before you sleep can also influence the quality of sleep you get. If you do an intense activity just before you sleep, your body is unable to rest well and go through the motions of repair and recovery. It is wiser to do a light activity close to bedtime. Furthermore, it is often good to ingest protein just before bed, as this helps to trigger the release of HGH, which stimulates repair and growth. A caseins protein powder shake would be the perfect candidate for a late-night snack. Your body undergoes the majority of its muscle repair and growth as you sleep. Not allowing it at least 8 hours to do so is going to completely negate any work you are doing in the gym. In order to see progress, you have to sleep.

Rest Days and Deload Weeks

Another important factor to take into account is rest days and deload weeks. As you start on your fitness journey, your body will require more rest days in your training routine in order to recover from all the new muscle growth and strain. You are undoubtedly already familiar with rest days, but you may not have heard of deload weeks before. Rest days are part of your regular training routine. You need to take at least 2 days of rest per week, either in between your active days or together after you have had 5 active days. Just like sleep, rest days are an essential part of preventing fatigue and allowing your muscles to recover and subsequently grow. If you want to see any progress at all, they are essential. They are also key in preventing overtraining.

Deload weeks are done for the same reasons you take rest days, but they are extended. A deload is a 'planned short period of recovery' (Samuels, 2018). They are usually done for a week, and the aim is to take your training slightly easier. This can be done through training less often or for shorter durations, training less intensely, doing a different type of training, or using lighter weights. You might be wondering why anyone would do this—
surely if you want to see gains, the key is to train harder. But just as rest days help to build muscle and strength, deload weeks are essential for achieving the same things. Deloads are also important for preventing overtraining. The idea is that you are giving your joints and ligaments a break, as well, which is key for preventing significant injuries. It also allows for a longer break than a few rest days, meaning your body has more time than usual to rest and recover. It can also be good for your mental health. Sometimes a less intense week is needed, as continued intensity and vigorous training can become overwhelming after a while. Adding deload weeks is important for seeing continual progress and avoiding plateaus.

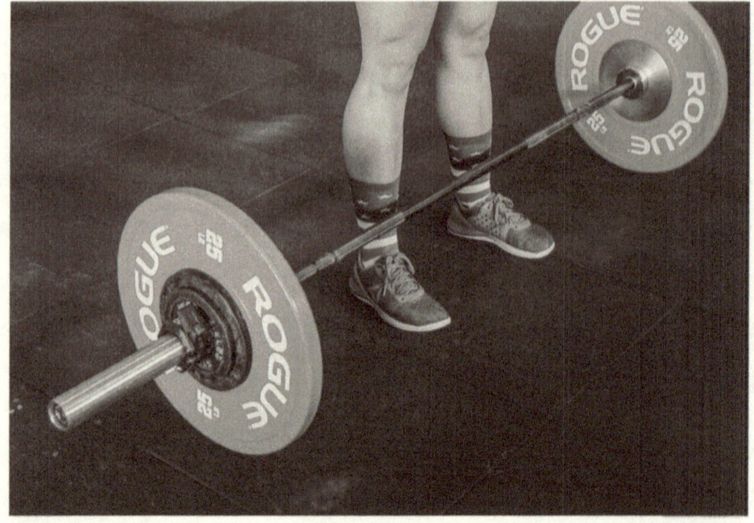

The first and most common form of deloading is to decrease your weights for the week. The general rule of thumb is to drop your weights to 40–60% of your one-rep max weight. You will do this for a whole week, with every exercise, while maintaining your usual workout routine. It may be tempting to up your reps while you do this, and continue to push yourself. But that would be completely undoing any good that is intended from a reload week—you need to take it slow. Otherwise, you may not be doing a deload week at all.

Another option is to keep your weight the same but reduce your volume. So, use the same weight for the same exercises but do half of the reps or sets you normally would. For example, let say you usually do a couple of sets of squats using 275 lbs for 5 reps. If you were deloading, you would only do 1 or 2 reps per set, or you would just do 1 set of 5 instead of a couple of sets. This technique is not as popular as the first I mentioned, but it does work well for some people. For example, competitive strength athletes tend to do this before a competition, as it allows them to train with the same heavy weights while still taking somewhat of a break.

The last method for deloading is to change up your training routine and do different exercises. This type of deloading is more beneficial for someone who is concerned with general fitness and strength, rather than someone who is competing or worried about high levels of performance (England, 2017). You could either switch to something similar, like a lower-intensity bodyweight circuit training. Or you could do something completely different!

You could focus on cardio-based mobility workouts like swimming or hiking throughout the week. This option is brilliant for those looking for a decent break for both their mental health and their muscles.

When you decide to deload is based upon a couple of factors, such as your overall goals, your training schedule, what level you are training at, and even how old you are. If you are training to compete or are at an advanced level of training, you would aim to take deload weeks less frequently. However, if you are training for general fitness and health, still a beginner or intermediate trainer, or older, you might want to take deload weeks more frequently.

There are a couple of signs that you should incorporate a deloading week. These will be similar to signs of overtraining. You may find you are getting weaker, and that you can no longer push yourself up in weights. This indicates that you are starting to overreach. It is also time for a deload week if you find that you are constantly struggling with energy when you go to work out or struggling with fatigue throughout the day. Another sign is that your joints are starting to get sore. It is natural to get a small injury from time to time, or find that your joints are sore now and then, especially after a particularly hard workout. However, if you are in constant aching pain when you work out, when you can't do one squat without your knees screaming at you, it is time to take a break in the form of a deload week.

There are three main deloading schedules that people tend to follow. The first is to do three weeks of training, followed by one deloading week. This is mainly used by professional or competing athletes in seasons, particularly the older ones. It can also be helpful when you are just starting out if your muscles and body are struggling with the new movement.

The second and most popular deload schedule is to take a deload week between every 6–8 weeks. A diverse range of people chose to do this one, everyone from professional athletes and competitive lifters, all the way to recreational lifters. This can be perfect if you are a recreational lifter who likes to travel occasionally, as it is the perfect schedule to incorporate a week of hiking around a new area, jogging on the beach, or skiing, as a few fun examples.

The last schedule is doing a deload every 12–16 weeks. This is used mostly by competitive lifters as well as intermediate or advanced recreational lifters.

The schedule you choose will depend entirely on your skill level and your goals. It is also important to listen to your body. If you do, you will know when it needs a break and when you should do less intense weeks. By playing around, you will find a deload schedule that works well for you.

Active Release Therapy

Rest and recovery is all about taking care of your muscles and your body, and another way to do that is through physical therapy methods such as active release therapy (ART). Active release therapy is a type of massage therapy performed both by physiotherapists and chiropractors. It has been around for about 30 years. It is a form of non-invasive manual therapy that uses a combination of manipulation and movement to correct soft-tissue restrictions that cause pain or issues with mobility while you are trying to be active (Santos-Longhurst, 2018).

Soft tissue issues can be caused either by acute injury or overuse injuries. Acute injuries are caused by sudden trauma, for example, falls, blows, or twists to the body. This can be a wrist or ankle sprain caused by bad form during a lift. Overuse injuries occur when an exercise is repeated often, and the body doesn't have sufficient time to heal in between (Mulcahey, 2020). Both of these are very real risks when you are weightlifting a few times a week and pushing yourself in order to see progress. Active release therapy can help to fix both of these types of injury.

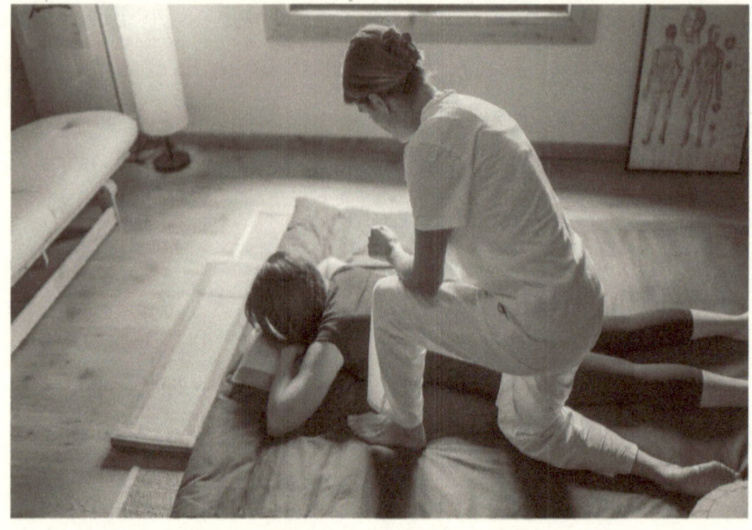

Many athletes and weightlifters use some form of physical therapy for maintenance. It is essential if you are suffering from a particular injury, however, it can also be helpful for preventing injuries by allowing increased flexibility and range of movement. Active release therapy is a brilliant method for removing any restrictions in your body, caused either by overuse, acute or chronic pain. It is essentially like a massage, but with motion and stretching. The therapist will instruct you to position your tissue so that it is active. They will then apply tension and instruct you to lengthen your muscle. The combination of tension and motion will be applied to several different areas, until you feel release. It can treat problems with your muscles, your ligaments, your tendons, and your nerves.

There are a number of different therapies that can be used to treat any injuries or soreness, as well as increase your functionality when you train. Many of these also treat soft tissue and are similar to active release therapy. One of the most popular therapies is deep tissue massage. This is very similar to active release therapy, as it combines pressure with active movement to release tension. However, deep tissue massage usually focuses on one area while ART can focus on multiple areas. Another method is called rolfing, which focuses mostly on manipulating and stretching your soft tissue in order to improve your posture and your spinal alignment. Graston technique massage has similar aims to ART, however, the therapist will use instruments instead of their hands to mobilize the tissue. Lastly, there is dry needling. This is when needles are pushed into the skin to release the tightness in your muscles. They push these needles into 'trigger points.' These are hard knots in your muscles that can cause stiffness and pain. The needle stimulates the trigger point, and the pain and stiffness release (Santos-Longhurst, 2018).

There are a number of benefits that come from active release therapy, whether or not you are suffering from an injury. It benefits the muscles, as it increases blood flow throughout the body, allowing for better pumps in the gym. This increased blood flow is also excellent for helping the muscles to grow in both strength and mass. It also allows for greater flexibility, which in turn helps with your range of motion and functionality while you lift (Yeun, 2017). In addition to treating injuries, active release therapy can also help to prevent them. Incorporating things like active release therapy into your routine ensures that your body is fully prepared and protected for any workout that you throw at it.

When you experience an injury, no matter how seemingly small or inconsequential, it is important to tend to it as quickly as possible. While many of these can be avoided by rest days, once you have an injury to a joint or a muscle, you will likely always feel it there. Physical therapies are essential for making sure these injuries are not holding you back as you continue on your fitness journey. Furthermore, many of these therapies help to improve general fitness, as well as your weightlifting training. They are great ways to make sure that your body is continually functioning at its peak and that your muscles are free of as much pain and tension as physically possible. They are an essential kind of maintenance that enables you to keep pushing your hardest when you are at the gym.

The time that you give your body to rest in between workouts is just as important as the workouts themselves. If you are continually pushing your body to its limits without giving it proper rest and care, it is going to start failing and breaking down. You only have one body in this life and you need to look after it. Furthermore, you are not going to see the progress you want if you do not rest. If your body doesn't have time to repair, it does not have time to build muscle and strength. Getting sleep, allowing for rest days and reload weeks, and active release therapy are not just suggestions or add ons for your workouts. They should be an essential part of your routine and fitness journey.

CONCLUSION

———— ◆◇◆ ————

The key to maximizing your workouts is knowledge. It is about understanding your body and how it responds to certain macronutrients, and why you need them to achieve your peak level of fitness. It is about understanding how to develop your workouts depending on what your goals are, how to incorporate cardio into your routine, and how to use supplements to push yourself to your limits. The biggest problem people have is not knowing exactly what they need to do. It is no longer as simple as picking up a magazine or looking up some opinions online—there is so much information that you would never know where to start!

But you no longer need to worry. Everything you need to know has been condensed into this book, and you no longer need to search. Depending on what your goals are, you can customize your workout routine and lifestyle accordingly. If your goal is general fitness, losing body fat, and gaining muscle, you can use a combination of the training styles. If you are focusing on the aesthetic progress you are making, you can do mainly hypertrophy workouts, adding in strength, endurance, and speed and agility workouts as you see fit. If you are looking to become strong, you can focus mainly on strength workouts.

You can add your preferred cardio, whether it is fasted or post-workout. Depending on where you are starting, you have three different general workout splits to choose from, and more variation within those three categories. If you have no experience, you can start as a beginner. If you have years of experience, you can start as an intermediate. You can decide which supplements best suit your goals, and when your workouts start to feel repetitive, there are a variety of ways you can mix them up to challenge your muscles again.

This book is not something you will read through once and forget about, it is a guide that you will keep coming back to throughout your journey in order to keep working harder and to keep your body challenged. You might try something and find it helpful, but not conducive to your goals or your motivation. Then you can come back, and try something else. This will be your bible for fitness and health—the book that you rely on to guide you and keep you going. Using these tips and tricks, you will see progress in weeks, and significant changes to your body and your fitness levels within months. It will start immediately, but it is also something you want to maintain going forward. This is not a fad diet or a 30-day fitness plan designed to "slim your waist and give you abs!" This book teaches you how to make fitness, weightlifting, and training a lifestyle. It makes it something that you can sustain because it is enjoyable and because you will always see the positive impacts on your life.

Now that you have these tools at your disposal, all you need to do is start. Sometimes this can feel like the hardest part, either because you have never done this before, or because you've tried dozens of different workout plans and none of them worked. But I can guarantee that with this book, this will be the last time you have to start from the beginning. The first day is always the hardest, so doesn't it make it easier to start this journey knowing that this is the last first day you'll have? The last first day of trying to change your eating habits to fit your fitness. The last first day of struggling through a new workout routine.

This book is so comprehensive, you will never have to try anything else. Sit down and figure out your workout routine, write it out. Factor in your cardio, and whether you plan to include other forms of training styles, such as endurance training or speed and agility training. Stock up on the foods and supplements that are going to help you through this journey. Completely prepare yourself for the weeks and months ahead so that doing the training comes easily and you don't hit up against preventable road blocks. And have fun!

If you have enjoyed this book and found it helpful don't forget to leave a review on Amazon! Now that you have finished, the only thing between you and your best self is the motivation to start. It just takes making the decision to change, to do better.

Once you have done that, it gets easier all the time. And even the smallest changes make a big difference. Start now—or later today, or tomorrow—but start soon. All that you have left to do is start!

A *Special* Gift to All of Our Readers!

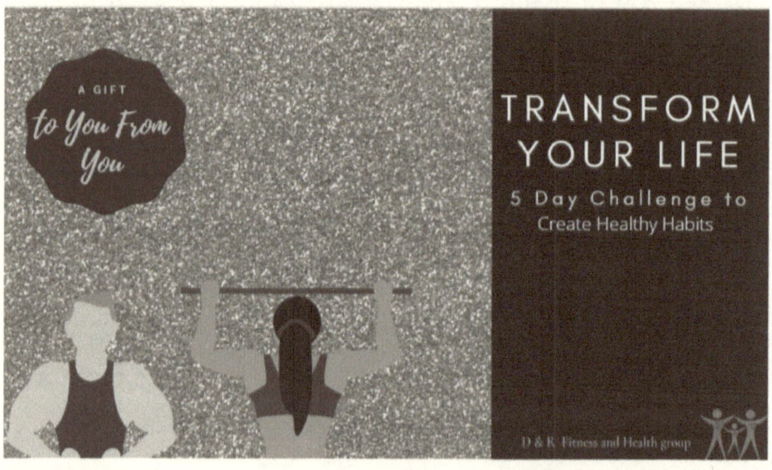

Included with your purchase of this book: You will receive a free copy of our "Transform Your life: 5 Day Challenge to Create Healthy habits" Which will take you day by day for 5 days to improve your life and your habits!

Don't miss out on this amazing opportunity to jump start the transformation of a life time.

Follow this link in order to claim your free copy today:

Drfitnessandhealthgroup.com

REFERENCES

Aceto, C. (2003). Chris Aceto's Instruction Book For Bodybuilding: Championship Bodybuilding. Morris Pub.

American Academy of Family Physicians. (2010). Hydration for Athletes. Family Doctor. https://familydoctor.org/athletes-theimportance-of-good-hydration/#:~:text=Good%20hydration%20means%20getting%20the

American College of Sports Medicine. (2009). Progression Models in Resistance Training for Healthy Adults. Medicine & Science in Sports & Exercise, 41(3), 687–708. https://doi.org/10.1249/mss.0b013e3181915670

Arrano, J. (2014). Weight lifter [Image]. In Unsplash. https://unsplash.com/photos/WSarPk6E5Fg

Baur, J. (2011). Drop Sets: What They Are and How to Use Them in Your Workout. STACK. https://www.stack.com/a/drop-sets-what-they-are-and-how-touse-them-in-yourworkout#:~:text=Drop%20sets%20increase%20muscle%20size

Bjarnadottir, A. (2017). How Drinking More Water Can Help You Lose Weight. Healthline. https://www.healthline.com/nutrition/drinking-water-helpswith-weight-loss

BlenderBottle Trainer Team. (2019). 2 Secrets To Grow Your Glutes. Blender Bottle Blog. https://blog.blenderbottle.com/2secrets-to-grow-your-glutes#:~:text=Tip%20%232%20%2D%20Mind%20to%20Muscle%20Connection&text=It%20is%20so%20important%20to

Boly, J. (2017). Supersets Explained: Benefits, Programming, and More. BarBend. https://barbend.com/supersets/

Boly, J. (2021). 3 Reasons Why You Should Perform Cardio After Lifting. BarBend. https://barbend.com/cardio-afterlifting/

Campbell, C., Prince, D., Braun, M., Applegate, E., & Casazza, G. A. (2008). Carbohydrate-Supplement Form and Exercise Performance. International Journal of Sports Nutrition and Exercise Metabolism, 18(2), 179–190. https://doi.org/10.1123/ijsnem.18.2.179

Carter, A. (2019). Do Multivitamins Work? The Surprising Truth. Healthline. https://www.healthline.com/nutrition/domultivitamins-work#ingredients

Chang, J. (2021). Swimming Laps [Image]. In Unsplash. https://unsplash.com/photos/N3VEiHD8Sec

Chen, R. (2018). Sugar and Weight Loss: How Sugar Affects Your Weight Loss Goals. Suspro Foods. https://www.susprofoods.com/blogs/news/sugar-and-weightloss-how-sugar-affects-your-weight-loss-goals

Chertoff, J. (2019). Muscular Hypertrophy and Your Workout. Healthline; Healthline Media. https://www.healthline.com/health/muscularhypertrophy#definition

Chertoff, J. (2020). Progressive Overload: What It Is, Examples, and Tips. Healthline. https://www.healthline.com/health/progressive-overload

Clark, B. C., Mahato, N. K., Nakazawa, M., Law, T. D., & Thomas, J. S. (2014). The Power of the Mind: the Cortex as a Critical Determinant of Muscle Strength/Weakness. Journal of Neurophysiology, 112(12), 3219–3226. https://doi.org/10.1152/jn.00386.2014

Cleveland Clinic. (2014). Carbohydrates. Cleveland Clinic. https://my.clevelandclinic.org/health/articles/15416carbohydrates

Cleveland Clinic. (2016). From Head to Toe: The Benefits of a Cardio Workout. Health Essentials from Cleveland Clinic; https://health.clevelandclinic.org/head-toe-benefits-cardioworkout-infographic/

Comite, F. (2013). Why You Should Avoid Carbs at Bedtime. Men's Health. https://www.menshealth.com/nutrition/a19539980/avoidcarbs-at-bedtime/#:~:text=When%20insulin%20is%20present%20because

Conscious Design. (2010). Deep Tissue Massage [Image]. In Unsplash. https://unsplash.com/photos/J16LdoIsRJM

Cronkleton, E. (2012). Warmup Exercises: 6 Ways to Get Warmed Up Before a Workout. Healthline. https://www.healthline.com/health/fitness-exercise/warm-upexercises#benefits

Culp, A. (2015). The Power of Vitamins in Athletics. Training & Conditioning. https://training-conditioning.com/article/thepower-ofvitamins/#:~:text=Most%20important%20to%20focus%20on

De Hamer, R. (2020). Treadmills [Image]. In Unsplash. https://unsplash.com/photos/pCT8ag1o3nU

DeYoung, M. (2015). Lemon Chicken [Image]. In Unsplash. https://unsplash.com/photos/mjcJ0FFgdWI

England, J. (2017). Deload Weeks: Everything You Need to Know on How to Deload. Muscle & Strength. https://www.muscleandstrength.com/articles/how-to-deload

Freitas, V. (2019). Lower weights [Image]. In Unsplash. https://unsplash.com/photos/WSarPk6E5Fg

Freitas, V. (2020). Adding Weights [Image]. In Unsplash. https://unsplash.com/photos/HG6aAf79Q5E

Gomez, A. (2016). Is Weight Loss Really 80 Percent Diet and 20 Percent Exercise? Women's Health. https://www.womenshealthmag.com/weightloss/a19982520/weight-loss-80-percent-diet-20-percentexercise/

Griffiths, A. (2019). Hypertrophy [Image]. In Unsplash. https://unsplash.com/photos/XW47yQNE0TQ

Grinnell, J. (2019). 10 Keys to Train for Endurance. Muscle & Fitness. https://www.muscleandfitness.com/workouts/workouttips/10-tips-endurance-training/

Harris-Fry, N. (2018). Casein Protein Basics: What Is It, What Are The Benefits And What Are The Side Effects? Coach.

https://www.coachmag.co.uk/supplements/7033/casein-proteinbasics-what-is-it-what-are-the-benefits-and-what-are-the-side

Harvard Health. (2018). Vitamins and Minerals. Help Guide. https://www.helpguide.org/harvard/vitamins-and-minerals.htm#:~:text=Vitamins%20and%20minerals%20are%2 0considered

Heyer, A. (2019). Forced Reps: Going Heavy! Bodybuilding. https://www.bodybuilding.com/fun/andy1.htm#:~:text=A%2 0r ep%20is%20considered%20%22forced

Holmes, M. (2019). Box Jump [Image]. In Unsplash. https://unsplash.com/photos/wy_L8W0zcpI

Huizen, J. (2018). 6 Reasons Why Drinking Water can Help you to Lose Weight. Www.medicalnewstoday.com. https://www.medicalnewstoday.com/articles/322296#sixreasons-why-drinking-water-may-help-you-lose-weight

International Sport Science Association. (2019). Does Lack of Sleep Hinder Muscle Growth or Performance? International Sport Science Association Online | ISSA. https://www.issaonline.com/blog/index.cfm/2018/does-lack-ofsleep-hinder-muscle-growth#:~:text=What%20researchers%20discovered%20was%2 0that

Johnson, K. (2018). Mind to Muscle [Image]. In Unsplash. https://unsplash.com/photos/Yi-4X9ZJU6Y

Kassel, G. (2019). Are There Really Any Benefits to Doing Fasted Cardio? Shape. https://www.shape.com/fitness/tips/what-is-fasted-cardiobenefits

Krzysztofik, M., Wilk, M., Wojdała, G., & Gołaś, A. (2019). Maximizing Muscle Hypertrophy: A Systematic Review of

Advanced Resistance Training Techniques and Methods. International Journal of Environmental Research and Public Health, 16(24),. https://doi.org/10.3390/ijerph16244897

Lavie, C. J., Arena, R., Swift, D. L., Johannsen, N. M., Sui, X., Lee, D., Earnest, C. P., Church, T. S., O'Keefe, J. H., Milani, R. V., & Blair, S. N. (2015). Exercise and the Cardiovascular System. Circulation Research, 117(2), 207–219. https://doi.org/10.1161/circresaha.117.305205

Lecompte, M. (2016). Abs Are Made in the Kitchen: The Rules You Need to Follow. Doctors Health Press. https://www.doctorshealthpress.com/food-and-nutritionarticles/abs-kitchen-rules/

Lyfe Fuel. (2019). Protein Powder [Image]. In Unsplash. https://unsplash.com/photos/phY30gaxqS8

M Club. (2017). The Pros and Cons of Pre-workout Supplements. M Club Spa and Fitness. https://mclubspaandfitness.co.uk/the-pros-and-cons-of-preworkout-supplements/#:~:text=The%20positives%20to%20using%20a%20pre%2Dworkout%20are%3A&text=Improves%20focus

Maragos, A. (2017). Bodybuilder [Unsplash]. In Unsplash. https://unsplash.com/photos/Yi-4X9ZJU6Y

Mayoclinic. (2019). Strength training: Get stronger, leaner, healthier. Mayo Clinic; https://www.mayoclinic.org/healthylifestyle/fitness/in-depth/strength-training/art-20046670 Medicine Plus. (2021). Nutrition and Athletic Performance. Medicine plus Medical Encyclopedia. https://medlineplus.gov/ency/article/002458.htm#:~:text=N%2 0utrition%20can%20help%20enhance%20athletic

Moqadam, S. (2019). Endurance Training [Image]. In Unsplash. https://unsplash.com/photos/pFVaARBtyXk

Msipa, N. (2019). Drinking Water [Image]. In Unsplash. https://unsplash.com/photos/OREidaPKnaA

Mulcahey, M. (2020). Sprains, Strains and Other Soft-Tissue Injuries. OrthoInfo. https://orthoinfo.aaos.org/en/diseases-conditions/sprains-strains-and-other-soft-tissueinjuries/#:~:text=Soft%2Dtissue%20injuries%20fall%20into

Nieścioruk, A. (2019). Vitamins [Image]. In Unsplash. https://unsplash.com/photos/hWzrJsS8gwI

Noonan, R. (2019). The Bakery. In Unsplash. https://unsplash.com/photos/6d5I1-gixyU

Opler, L. (2019). The Mind-Muscle Connection. Www.acefitness.org. https://www.acefitness.org/education-andresources/lifestyle/blog/7388/the-mind-muscle-connection/

Ottinger, C. (2019). Eccentrics and Growth. The Muscle PhD. https://themusclephd.com/eccentrics-and-growth/#:~:text=Eccentrics%20and%20Research&text=A%20 muscle%20can%20produce%20anywhere

Piedmont Healthcare. (2019). Why is Protein Important in your Diet? Piedmont.org. https://www.piedmont.org/livingbetter/why-is-protein-important-in-your-diet

Pullen, C. (2017). 7 Ways Sleep Can Help You Lose Weight. Healthline; Healthline Media. https://www.healthline.com/nutrition/sleep-and-weight-loss

Quinn, E. (2007). Why Carbohydrates Are Important for Exercise. Verywell Fit; https://www.verywellfit.com/howcarbohydrate-provides-energy-3120661

Rachel Reiff Ellis. (2019). Surprising Reasons to Get More Sleep. WebMD;
https://www.webmd.com/sleepdisorders/benefits-sleep-more

Redl, A. (2017). Sprinting In Vienna [Image]. In Unsplash. https://unsplash.com/photos/d3bYmnZ0ank

Reid Health. (2017). Carbohydrates 101: The Benefits of Carbohydrates. Reid Health.
https://www.reidhealth.org/blog/carbohydrates-101-thebenefits-of-carbohydrates#:~:text=Carbohydrates%20are%20your%20body

Richey, B. (2018). Everything You Need to Know About Speed Training. Breaking Muscle.
https://breakingmuscle.com/fitness/everything-you-need-toknow-about-speed-training

Robertson, R. (2018). 13 Benefits of Taking Fish Oil. Healthline Media; https://www.healthline.com/nutrition/13benefits-of-fish-oil

Saini, V. (2020, July 12). 6 Ways To Improve Your MindMuscle Connection. Generation Iron Fitness & Bodybuilding Network.
https://generationiron.com/improve-your-mindmuscle-connection/

Salter, P. (2016). Your Guide to Intra-Workout Carbohydrates. Bodybuilding.com.
https://www.bodybuilding.com/content/your-guide-to-intraworkout-carbohydrates.html

Samuels, M. (2018). Deloading 101: What Is a Deload and How Do You Do It? Breaking Muscle.
https://breakingmuscle.com/fitness/deloading-101-what-is-adeload-and-how-do-you-do-it

Santos-Longhurst, A. (2018). 10 Active Release Technique Benefits. Healthline. https://www.healthline.com/health/activerelease-technique

Schepis, J. (2019). Upper Back Training: 4 Tips to Enhance Your Mind Muscle Connection & Growth! JPS Health & Fitness. https://www.jpshealthandfitness.com.au/upper-backtraining-4-tips-to-enhance-your-mind-muscle-connectiongrowth/

Scheumeier, S. (2020). Fresh Vegetable Produce [Image]. In Unsplash. https://unsplash.com/photos/4R1YpmGO52I

Schinetsky, R. (2019). Pros and Cons of Fasted Cardio. Nutrex Research. https://www2.nutrex.com/blog/pros-and-cons-offasted-cardio/

Shaw, A. (2020). Stretching [Image]. In Unsplash. https://unsplash.com/photos/qB3s3bTE8_0

Simone, M. (2013). 5 Muscle-Shocking Methods you Forgot. Men's Journal. https://www.mensjournal.com/health-fitness/5muscle-shocking-methods-you-forgot-all-about/

Sol, A. (2019). Sleeping [Image]. In Unsplash. https://unsplash.com/photos/OREidaPKnaA String, J. (2014). Pre-Workout Buzz: A Look Into Pre Workout Supplementation. Hunt Fitness. https://www.kylehuntfitness.com/the-pre-workout-buzz/

Sweat. (2019). How To Break Through A Workout Plateau. SWEAT. https://www.sweat.com/blogs/fitness/workoutplateau#:~:text=As%20your%20body%20adapts%2C%20exerc ises

Thomas, M. H., & Burns, S. P. (2019). Increasing Lean Mass and Strength: A Comparison of High Frequency Strength Training to Lower Frequency Strength Training. International Journal of Exercise Science, 9(2), 159–167.

Tinsley, G. (2017). 7 Benefits of High-Intensity Interval Training (HIIT). Healthline; https://www.healthline.com/nutrition/benefits-of-hiit

Tinsley, G. (2018). Whey Protein Isolate vs Concentrate: What's The Difference? Healthline. https://www.healthline.com/nutrition/whey-protein-isolate-vsconcentrate#TOC_TITLE_HDR_2

Warner, J. (2014). Protein Powder: Everything You Need to Know. Coaching Mag; https://www.coachmag.co.uk/nutrition/supplements/3839/prot ein-powder-a-comprehensive-guide-for-beginners

Women's Sport Medical Centre. (2018). What Are the Warning Signs & Symptoms of Overtraining? Hospital for Special Surgery. https://www.hss.edu/conditions_overtraining.asp

Wunsch, K., Kasten, N., & Fuchs, R. (2017). The Effect of Physical Activity on Sleep Quality, Well-being, and Affect in Academic Stress Periods. Nature and Science of Sleep, Volume 9, 117–126. https://doi.org/10.2147/nss.s132078

Yetman, D. (2020). Endurance Vs. Stamina: Differences and Tips to Improve Both. Healthline. https://www.healthline.com/health/exercise-fitness/endurancevs-stamina

Yeun, Y.-R. (2017). Effectiveness of Massage Therapy on the Range of Motion of the shoulder: A Systematic Review and Meta-analysis. Journal of Physical Therapy Science, 29(2), 365–369. https://doi.org/10.1589/jpts.29.365